Reimagining Social Medicine from the South

Reimagining Social Medicine from the South

Abigail H. Neely

Duke University Press
Durham and London
2021

© 2021 Duke University Press. All rights reserved.
Printed and bound by CPI Group (UK) Ltd, Croydon, CR0 4YY
Designed by Drew Sisk
Project editor: Susan Albury
Typeset in Portrait Text and Helvetica by Copperline Book Services

Library of Congress Cataloging-in-Publication Data
Names: Neely, Abigail H., [date] author.
Title: Reimagining social medicine from the South /
Abigail H. Neely.
Description: Durham: Duke University Press, 2021. | Includes
bibliographical references and index.
Identifiers: LCCN 2020047368 (print)
LCCN 2020047369 (ebook)
ISBN 9781478013365 (hardcover)
ISBN 9781478014270 (paperback)
ISBN 9781478021582 (ebook)
Subjects: LCSH: Social medicine—South Africa. | Community
health services—South Africa. | Health promotion—South Africa. |
Primary health care—South Africa.
Classification: LCC RA418.3. S6 N44 2021 (print) |
LCC RA418.3. S6 (ebook) | DDC 362.10968—dc23
LC record available at https: //lccn.loc.gov/2020047368
LC ebook record available at https: //lccn.loc.gov/2020047369

Duke University Press gratefully acknowledges the Department
of Geography and the Associate Dean of the Social Sciences at
Dartmouth College, who provided funds toward the production
of this book.

Cover art: Illustration and design by Drew Sisk. Source images:
Sergii Telesh / Alamy Stock Photo (beetroot); typhoid map
from an outbreak in the Ngwagane community in South Africa,
1951 Annual Report, SAB, GES vol. 1917, ref. 46/32.

For Allie

CONTENTS

On a sticky July day in 2008, I found myself sitting on the edge of a white, modern sofa in the immaculate living room of a brownstone in Brooklyn Heights. Perched on an ottoman across the room was Dr. Jack Geiger, an academic clinician and one of the best-known proponents of social medicine. Social medicine is a branch of medicine that combines an attention to the social determinants of health (often understood as poverty) and the biology of disease. I had come to talk with Dr. Geiger about the five months he had spent in South Africa while he was in medical school more than fifty years earlier learning about community-oriented primary care (COPC), a brand of social medicine that I would come to learn was associated with an international movement to extend primary health care to the world's poorest people. Back in the United States on a short break from my fieldwork in South Africa, I stopped in New York for a couple of quick interviews. This was my first.

I had spent the previous six months in the rural, mountainous, Zulu-speaking area of South Africa, locally known as Pholela, investigating relationships between health and landscape and how they did and did not change between the 1930s and the present. I was drawn to this place in part because Pholela had been the site of a state-funded-and-run health center (later in coordination with the University of Natal and the Rockefeller Foundation). I took this to mean that there was a good chance of a strong archival record, which I presumed was important for understanding change over time. Only after I arrived did I discover that the Pholela Community Health Centre (PCHC) had an impressive global reputation. Indeed, historians and social medicine experts in academic and practitioner spheres remember it with great admiration.[1] I had planned to do a project that would reframe understandings of health and landscape from the perspective of Pholela and its people. Because I was so focused on telling a story *from* Pholela, I originally imagined that the PCHC, its program, and its staff would be only minor players. But even within just the first few months of research, it became clear that the PCHC was important to life, livelihoods, and health in Pholela (not to mention to social medicine more broadly), and further, that it would play an important role in the story I would tell.

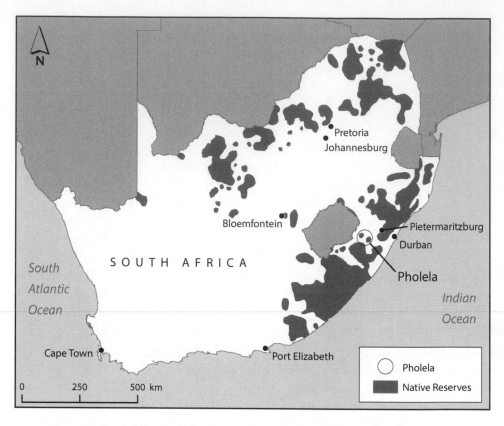

Figure P.1 South Africa in 1940 when the Pholela Community Health Center was established. Map created by Jonathan W. Chipman, Citrin GIS Lab, Dartmouth College.

As I began to look for former staff members to talk to, I quickly learned that my search would be more difficult than I imagined. All of the doctors had long since left South Africa, and almost everyone who had worked at the PCHC had passed away. It was in this search that I came across Dr. Geiger's name. I knew only that he was American and that he had spent some time in Pholela as a medical student. I found Dr. Geiger's email address and sent him a message. Remarkably, he responded, putting me in touch with a few other US-based people who had some experience with the PCHC. He also agreed to meet me for an interview.

Dr. Geiger was a well-respected activist known for extending health care to people living in poverty. He was a founding member of a number of advocacy groups, including Physicians for Human Rights, which won the 1997 Nobel Peace Prize.[2] He was also a member of the United States National Academy

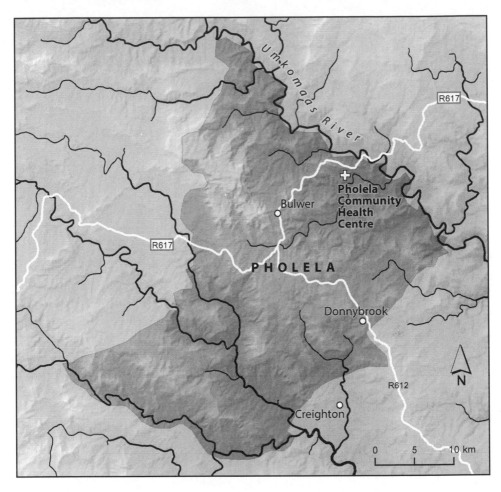

Figure P.2 Map of Pholela. Created by Jonathan W. Chipman, Citrin GIS Lab, Dartmouth College.

of Medicine and the Institute of Medicine, which awarded him the Gustav O. Lienhard Award for Advancement of Health Care for his work with COPC. As I fought my way through New York City traffic to visit Dr. Geiger, I had plenty of time to wonder why this world-famous doctor was willing to take time out of a Saturday afternoon to talk with me, a PhD student in the seemingly unre- lated discipline of geography.

As anyone who had met him will attest, Dr. Geiger had tremendous energy and enthusiasm, and this showed the instant he opened the door. After we shook hands, he briskly walked me to his living room, where he asked if I would like a coffee or something else to drink. When I said I'd love a glass of water, he replied that he was going to brew some strong coffee because he knew he needed it for the conversation we were about to have. It was at that moment that I got the first hint that Dr. Geiger was as nervous about our meeting as I was.

I had barely begun to explain my project and the research I'd been conducting when Dr. Geiger jumped in and asked about the people in Pholela and how they were doing. He didn't ask after anyone in particular; he wanted to know how the community was, how health was, and how the transition out of apartheid had been for the communities and families with whom the health center had worked most closely. Apartheid was the decades-long period of minority rule marked by oppressive policies of segregation and discrimination that began only a decade before Dr. Geiger went to Pholela and ended in the early 1990s when Nelson Mandela was elected president. As I described life in Pholela, Dr. Geiger sat balanced on the edge of the ottoman, rapt with attention. He wanted to know anything I could tell him. He asked about the health center, but his real interests lay in the lives and homesteads of Pholela's residents.

Our conversation shifted to Dr. Geiger's experiences in Pholela. In 1957, he was a medical student at Case Western Reserve. Before medical school, he had a career as a science journalist and participated in what is today termed anti-racism work. This led him to an interest in the possibilities of medicine for social justice. He heard about the Institute for Family and Community Health (IFCH) at the University of Natal's Medical School in Durban. In this institute, a group of doctors, including Sidney and Emily Kark, the founders of the PCHC, had developed a training center for social medicine based on work they had begun in Pholela. Soon Geiger had secured funding and time off from school, and he was in South Africa learning about COPC.

Telling his story, Dr. Geiger fast-forwarded a few years to the 1960s. He was a professor at Harvard Medical School and it was Freedom Summer (1964). He was involved with an organization that provided free medical care to activists headed to Mississippi to register black voters. As he traveled around the state and saw how many people lived without health care, he began to think about what a health care intervention for people living in poverty might look like. His mind immediately returned to South Africa.

After that summer, Geiger got in touch with Sargent Shriver, who had taken charge of planning President Lyndon Johnson's War on Poverty through the Office of Economic Opportunity. Geiger knew that the government was already hard at work on other aspects of the program and wanted to offer some ideas about the health component. As we sat in his Brooklyn brownstone, he told me about a two-hour meeting he had with Shriver in which all that he had learned and experienced in Pholela poured out. Shriver took pages and pages of notes on a yellow-lined legal pad, as Geiger offered the Pholela Community Health Centre's brand of COPC as a model for health care delivery among economically disadvantaged people in the United States. Once he had finished describing the model, he offered a plan to develop two health centers—one in the Mississippi Delta, where he had spent the summer, and one in Boston, where he lived and worked. Geiger estimated that he would need $30,000 (about $250,000 in 2020 terms) to develop an initial plan for the health centers. Geiger recalls that Shriver replied, "Nonsense, you'll take $300,000 and you'll have the health centers up and running within a year."

With colleagues at Tufts University, which had agreed to provide institutional support, Geiger created the Columbia Point Community Health Center (now called the Geiger-Gibson Community Health Center) in a public housing project in Boston and the Delta Community Health Center in Mound Bayou, Mississippi, an independent Black community founded by former slaves. These establishments did more than function as clinics; they became access points for social services and hubs of community organizing for the people and places they serve. They were designed with the goal of absolute empowerment, to help raise people out of poverty and to end ill health. These two health centers then became the models for a network of more than eight thousand community health centers in the United States that provide care for over twenty million underserved individuals to this day.[3] As he finished the story, Dr. Geiger repeated that it was the Pholela Community Health Center that the War on Poverty had to thank. Moreover, he said, millions of Americans are indebted to this remote place where COPC was born for their health care and for access to social services.

The United States is not alone in benefiting from the social medicine program developed in Pholela. As work became untenable under apartheid, the doctors at the PCHC left South Africa to continue their work elsewhere. Many of the doctors were Jewish and, inspired by the Kibbutz movement, emigrated to Israel, bringing the COPC model with them. In the 1960s and 1970s, they managed to reorient Israel's health care system around community health centers.[4] Others found jobs in places like the United States, Canada, Colombia, and Uganda. As these doctors traveled, they brought COPC with them. It became one of the most important models of social medicine worldwide in the second half of the twentieth century.[5]

In the late 1950s, the last medical director of the PCHC, John Bennet, along with George Gale, a prominent doctor and social medicine proponent, left

Pholela and South Africa for Uganda and the Makerere University Medical School. Makerere was one of the premier institutions of higher learning in Africa in the 1950s and 1960s, and at the university these two South Africans developed a curriculum centered around "community public health," "which took into account traditional and cultural values of the local community"; this was COPC.[6] Thanks to this focus on social medicine at the country's only medical school, COPC remained central to health care in Uganda, to the benefit of much of the population, until Idi Amin's regime came to power in the 1970s, when many of the doctors and public health experts trained at Makerere University left the country.

In spite of COPC's relatively brief heyday in Uganda, universities, including Makerere University, have long been key to its success globally. In South Africa, the Karks and their team trained a number of doctors, and once those doctors left, they took up positions at universities around the world teaching others how to practice COPC. In 1959, the Karks themselves went to Israel to help set up what would come to be known as the Department of Public Health and Community Medicine at Hebrew University (now the Braun School) as part of a three-year WHO-funded program. Once the program was established, they stayed and Sidney chaired the department until he retired in 1980. To this day, the Braun School educates people from around the world in the principles and practices of COPC, helping to extend its reach. For example, Gcina Radebe, a recent district manager of health for the area including Pholela, and current KwaZulu-Natal provincial head of primary health care, received her MPH from Hebrew University, where she learned about the very COPC that was originally developed in what would become her home district. She then brought that back to the work she does in KwaZulu-Natal.[7]

Still others who had worked and trained in Pholela brought the ideas and techniques of social epidemiology—the study of social factors shaping health at the population scale—which was integral to health center practice in Pholela, to universities around the world. For example, John Cassel, the second medical director of the PCHC, moved from Durban, South Africa, to Chapel Hill, North Carolina, where he established and chaired the program in epidemiology at the University of North Carolina, with a focus on social epidemiology.[8] And in 1978, Sidney Kark was among the authors of the World Health Organization's Alma Ata Declaration on primary health care for all, based in part on ideas he first developed in Pholela.

The story I heard from Dr. Geiger and the stories I would hear a few days later from Mervyn Susser and Norm Scotch were the first of many stories about the history of COPC and the role of the PCHC that I would come to hear or read in the years that followed. In each case, these stories reinforced my first impressions from Dr. Geiger; this out-of-the-way place in this country, deep in the Southern Hemisphere, had an impact on the world far beyond what anyone expected.

The birth of COPC in Pholela and social medicine more generally is a well-known story. Yet in all of these truly remarkable stories, something was missing: the voices of Pholela's people and the stories of their lives. When I sat down with Dr. Geiger, he wanted to know about the *people* of Pholela. He wanted to know about their lives, their health, and their experiences since the PCHC had lost its funding in 1962. He knew how important they were to his life's work.

This is a book about social medicine, its possibilities, and its limitations, told through the lives and experiences of those people. It is not a book about the history of the PCHC, of COPC, or of social medicine more generally, at least not in any narrow sense. (And it is no longer a book about the relationships between health and landscape, though they do play a role.) It is first and foremost a book from Pholela. As such, this book offers a story of social medicine as developed and practiced by the PCHC and as experienced by the people who lived around it. It also offers stories of medicine practiced by traditional healers like *izangoma* and *izinyanga* and experienced by Pholela's residents.[9] All of these stories of doctors and izangoma, of health assistants and residents, of nutrients and witchcraft, are anchored in the lives and homes of Pholela's residents. Telling a story of social medicine from the home landscapes and lives—from the worlds—of Pholela's residents, offers important insight into what happened in Pholela, into the social medicine that began there and moved around the world, and into global health today.

As this book reveals, the history of social medicine isn't just a story of famous doctors and epidemiologists; it's a story of rural African peasants, vegetable gardens, nutrients, witchcraft, ancestors, healers, and more. To think about social medicine without these actors is to miss a big piece of the story. As I argue in this book, it is not possible to understand the global story of social medicine without understanding the lives of Pholela's residents, their homesteads, their health, and their worlds. Examining social medicine and health and healing from Pholela teaches much about the possibilities and limitations of this science and pushes for a more-than-human understanding of social life in health and healing.

ACKNOWLEDGMENTS

This is a book about how shifting a starting point changes both the stories we tell and how we understand the realities we inhabit. As a result, it seems appropriate that I start my thanks in Pholela, the place from which these stories come and the place that has forever shaped who I am as a scholar and a person. My first and biggest thanks go to Thokozile Nguse, who has been my key interlocutor for more than thirteen years now. I conducted all of the ethnographic research for this book with Thoko, who is equal parts sister, friend, research assistant, and sounding board. Her grace, wisdom, and humility inform all of the research and writing I have conducted, and I thank her not only for helping me understand and know this place, but for teaching me how to be in Pholela and in life more generally. Nonhlanhla Dlamini has been a wonderful friend, guide, and interlocutor from my earliest days in her community. More thanks go to Solani Shezi, Thabisile Dlamini, Lulu Sokhela, and Khanyisile Dlamini for all their companionship and introductions. I also owe a big thanks to Thoko's extended family, who have always given me a home in Pholela, and to the Phoswa family, who have done the same. Fieldwork can be grinding and tiring, but the chance to sit with, chat with, sing with, and marvel at all of my dear *gogos* has always put a smile on my face and reminded me why I do what I do. *Ngiyabonga kakhulu, bonke bagogo bam. Kakhulu.*

Beyond Pholela, Yvonne and Mike Lello have offered me a home away from home in Durban for fifteen years now. I can't imagine better surrogate parents. Cathy Connely and the late John Daniel also provided a warm home and fantastic conversation for me while in Durban. For many visits and adventures in Durban and Pholela and for years of great conversations and walks on the beachfront, a big thanks to Saskia Wustafeld. Barney and Faye Flett have provided countless meals and trips to the beach and the game park, all a welcome break from the research. In Pretoria, the late Koos and Marita Prinsloo gave me a warm home and some wonderful meals as I spent months in the archives. Susan and David Yuill have provided me a place to stay and much needed distraction in Johannesburg for years. They were my first entry to KZN and Gauteng fifteen years ago, and they remain the best hosts I know. In the early days, Chris Lello was often there too and up for a meal or a movie or a trip to the pub. In Bulwer, which has long been my home base in Pholela, I owe thanks to many friends who made life outside of research not just bearable, but fun. Thanks to Anne-Marie Assémat-Schmitt, Johan Smal, the late Dave and Linda Poval, the Rennies, Esther Alm, Pete Ablitt, Hans and Ria Fockens, the late Bruce McClunan, the late Les Pitt, and Sindey Dlamini. And a big thanks to Lauretta Grobler, who provides a warm bed and the most delicious meals every time I return.

A special thanks to those people and organizations in South Africa who helped me set up and conduct my research: Catherine Burns, Steve Reid, Malcolm Draper, Tim Quinlan, the Valley Trust, Gcina Radebe, Sister Sikhakhane, Dr. Gumede, the Pholela Community Health Centre, and the Turn Table Trust. Thanks to the librarians and archivists at the National Archives Repository in Pretoria, the Natal Archives Repository in Pietermaritzburg, the Historical Papers at the University of the Witwatersrand in Johannesburg, the Chief Directorate of Surveys and Mapping for South Africa in Cape Town, and the Killie Campbell Library in Durban.

As all scholars know, material support underlies all good ideas. For financial support, I thank the National Science Foundation, the Land Tenure Center at the University of Wisconsin–Madison, the John Sloan Dickey Center for International Understanding at Dartmouth, the Mellon Foundation, and the Burke Award from Dartmouth College. Many thanks to the Agrarian Studies Program at Yale, which gave me a year to think and write and an outstanding intellectual community in which to do so.

All good ideas are born from conversations with smart people. Put another way, the best scholarship is collective and I have a big collective to thank. The University of Wisconsin–Madison, and in particular the Geography Department, African history program, and Center for Culture, History, and Environment provided an incredibly generative space to begin this project. Many thanks go to Mitch Aso, Nick Bauch, Martha Bell, Dawn Biehler, Sarah Besky, Leif Brottem, Eric Carter, Chris Duvall, Nicole Eggers, Jake Fleming, Mara Goldman, Po-Yi Hung, Jess Krug, Chris Limburg, Dan Magaziner, Adam Mandleman, Hannah Nyala-West, Sig Peterson, Beth Stockbridge, and Yen-Chu Wang. I worked out many of the core ideas of the dissertation that preceded this book on long runs with Todd Dresser. My thanks go to him for his willingness to think with me and to slow down to a pace I could keep up with. Andrew Case and Amrys Williams taught me that you get to choose your family and that they can be smart interlocuters too. Finally, I owe much of the scholarly grounding in this book to conversations I've had with Alex Nading, who introduced me to medical anthropology (and a whole bunch of super-smart medical anthropologists) and continues to be one of my favorite people to think with.

At UW I had the good fortune to have some exceptional mentors. Many thanks go to Lisa Naughton, Neil Kodesh, and Claire Wendland for guiding me through my dissertation and beyond. A special thanks to Gregg Mitman, who, at my dissertation defense, pointed out that I had black-boxed social medicine. In many senses this book is a response to that realization. Another thanks to William Beinart, who advised my masters work at Oxford and welcomed me back to write for a term in graduate school. His unparalleled knowledge of South African history and his generosity helped me to become the scholar I am. Even before I had the good fortune to work with him, Bill Cronon taught me the importance of good writing, and good storytelling more specifically. I hope some of that teaching comes through here. My biggest thanks go to Matt Turner, the absolute best adviser a graduate student could ask for. Matt's commitment to ethical, engaged, creative, and rigorous scholarship offers both a challenge and a model, and his ability to mentor his students where they are to wherever they might end up is remarkable. I've talked this book through with Matt more times than anyone else and it has benefited tremendously from his smarts and generosity.

I feel lucky to have started my career at the University of Minnesota, where I found a group of tremendously smart colleagues who pushed my thinking in new directions. Many thanks go to Nikhil Anand, Bruce Braun, Susan Craddock, Vinay Gidwani, Jennifer Gunn, George Henderson, Brenda Kayzar, Reg Kunzel, Lorena Munoz, Abdi Samatar, Rachel Schurman, Martin Swobodzinski, and Dominique Tobbel. I spent a year as a fellow in the Agrarian Studies program at Yale, where I had the space and time to think and exposure to all sorts of new ideas. Special thanks go to Tom Fleischman, Karen Hebert, Tenzin Jinba, Jim Scott, and Shivi (Kalyanakrishnan Sivaramakrishnan).

The Geography Department at Dartmouth College is hands down the best place to work in academia. My colleagues are brilliant, generous, and committed to building a better world and a better university. It is a privilege and an honor to work and think with them. My thanks go to Luis Alvarez León, Mona Domosh, Treva Ellison, Coleen Fox, Frank Magilligan, Justin Mankin, Kelly Palmer, Darius Scott, Xun Shi, Jonathan Winter, and Richard Wright. Special thanks go to Susanne Freidberg and Chris Sneddon who read the first draft of my book manuscript and subsequent drafts of sections, offering invaluable feedback along the way. And a big thanks to Jonathan Chipman for not only being a great office neighbor, but also being a talented map maker who helped with the maps for this book. We've also been lucky at Dartmouth to have some pretty awesome human geography postdocs who have taught me a lot. Thanks to Kate Hall, Yui Hashimoto, Greta Marchesi, Garrett Nelson, and Brian Williams. More thanks go to brilliant colleagues across the university for thinking through ideas and just providing a good place to live and work. Thanks to Aimee Bahng, Sienna Craig, Reena Goldthree, Chelsey Kivland, Eng-Beng Lim, Anne Sosin, Craig Sutton, and George Trumbull.

Over the past few years I've had the good fortune to get to know brilliant interlocutors in geography, anthropology, African studies, and more. For teaching me, encouraging me, and thinking with me, many thanks go to Cal Biruk, Heidi Hausermann, Paul Jackson, Brian King, Becky Mansfield, and Laura Meek. For intellectual and general camaraderie in South Africa and back home over the years, my thanks go to Abigail Baim-Lance, Jessica Powers, and Liz Thornberry. Special thanks go to Julie Guthman, who flew across the country to spend three hours talking about the first version of my book manuscript and who offered valuable insight. This book is far stronger as a result of her brilliance. Thanks to Ramah McKay, who has offered so much on so many things I've thought about and pointed me to the best of anthropology since our early days at Minnesota, and to Keith Woodward, who has long been my sounding board for anything theory related and from whom I have learned so much. I was tremendously lucky to arrive at Dartmouth with Tish Lopez, who, over shouted questions and observations across the hallway in Fairchild and long text exchanges, has proven to be one of the smartest, most generous people I know. Her commitment to enacting a caring world through her research, teaching, and being is a model we should all follow. A last big thanks goes to Laura Ogden, who is not only a writer I aspire to be like, but who read two complete drafts of this book and, as I neared the end, reminded me that this is my book and I get to choose what it says and how. And then she cheered me to the finish line. A million thanks to all of you and many more.

Courtney Berger met with me once many years ago when I was in Durham to chat about an idea I had for a book. Since then, she has been an excellent shepherd for this project and the many forms it has taken, offering me expert advice and talking with me as I found my own way forward. Thanks to her, I had the good fortune of getting incredible feedback and engagement from four anonymous reviewers. What a lucky, lucky thing for a scholar. More thanks to Sandra Korn, who has gathered all the manuscript pieces and answered all my questions. And a big thanks to Rebecca Kohn for her editorial expertise on my first manuscript and to Aurora Chang for her copyediting work on the last. Last, portions of chapter 4 previously appeared as "Entangled Agencies: Rethinking Causality and Health in Political-Ecology," *Environment and Planning E: Nature and Space* (2020): doi.org/10.1177/2514848620943889, and have been significantly revised for this manuscript.

Writing a book, especially one based in long-term fieldwork conducted for extended stretches in a place that takes more than a day to get to, takes a lot. I've always said that the reason I can travel so far so often for so long is that I have such a wonderful family to come home to. Many thanks to my brothers Will and John Neely and to Justine, Rose, Koji, and Candace, who have always ensured that I have a home to come back to, and even some laughs. I'm also blessed with a bunch of cousins and an extended family, some of whom now live in Johannesburg. How lucky it is to have a home away from home thanks to Phoebe and James Boardman and William and Thomas. As I was writing the first draft of this book, I met Allie Breslaw and soon had the good fortune of being welcomed into the most wonderful extended Breslaw-DeSousa-Tharinger family. My life is so much richer and happier as a result of joining them.

I owe so much to my feminist parents, Christine Sullivan and John Neely, who raised their daughter to be smart, strong, and a tad rebellious. Just after I submitted this manuscript, my mom passed away suddenly and unexpectedly. The last text exchange I had with her was to tell her that Duke had agreed to send my book out for review. She was thrilled. The revisions I undertook were under a cloud of sadness, and my heart hurts because she is not here to hold this book in her hands, but I look forward to celebrating with my dad and maybe crying a little at her absence.

Luckily for me, the sadness of that loss has been tempered by tremendous joy. My biggest thanks go to Liam, who came with Allie, and who taught me that being a mom could be even more fun than writing a book. And now to Theo, who arrived just days after I got my book contract and whose unstoppable joy makes everything better. And finally, to Allie, who is the best partner, papa, home builder, project taker-oner, listener, and life maker I can imagine. He brings me cups of tea, takes the baby away when I need to write and don't want him to go, and keeps our home and family together when I'm off giving a talk, doing more research, tucked away writing, and much of the rest of the time too. He has made it so I can have a life that is rich and full of ideas and scholarship as well as love and fun. It is for this and so much more that I dedicate this book to him.

Telling the Story of Social Medicine from Pholela

One hot April afternoon in 2009, I sat with a remarkably healthy older Zulu-speaking woman in her garden in Pholela, South Africa. We were discussing common health concerns among her generation. Gogo (Grandma) Ngcobo had an impressive garden. In addition to maize, millet, and sorghum, she grew vegetables like spinach, green peppers, beetroot, and carrots. Organized in separate beds and planted in rows, Gogo Ngcobo's garden could have served as an advertisement for scientific management.

As we sat under a shady tree, she told me that the loss of "traditional" foods had led to hypertension and type 2 diabetes. In particular, she blamed the "new" store-bought maize meal people consumed in large quantities, claiming it was not as healthy as the maize meal made by people from their own corn. When maize meal is processed, she explained, "this little thing in the middle of the maize kernel is taken out," and the maize is ground without it. This little piece was important, Gogo told me, because it was the "healthy part."[1]

As conversations about health in 2009 were wont to do, Gogo's became a lament about the poor health of the "youth" (people between the ages of fifteen and thirty-five). While she acknowledged that the youth were suffering (and dying) from "these diseases" (often understood as a gloss for HIV/AIDS), she claimed that bad food was the reason the youth were so sick in the first place.[2] According to Gogo, young people in Pholela were getting sick because they had "weak blood." She blamed this weak blood on the consumption of "bad food" like commercial maize meal and cooking oil. Cooking oil, she explained, goes to the knees and makes them sore; even the smell makes her stomach "sad." She went on to say that undercooking and boiling (as opposed to frying) food

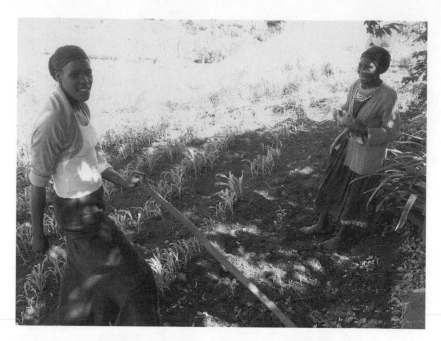

Figure I.1 Gogo Ngcobo with Thokozile in Gogo's garden. Photo by author.

from the garden is the healthiest option. This cooking method is important for preserving the food's "nutrients." "Nutrients are important because they help the blood to function well." And well-functioning blood is key for good health.

As I sat in the shade chatting with Gogo, I remembered one of my first visits to her garden. I had asked her to give me a tour. We ambled around and she showed me the grains and vegetables that she would later reap and eat and pointed with pride to the ornamental plants and trees she had received from her children working in distant cities. As we got to the middle of the garden, I pointed to a small, unfamiliar plant with long leaves and asked Gogo what it was called and what it was for. She looked at me and smiled, slightly embarrassed, "Oh that? It's nothing. It's just *intelezi*." Intelezi is the plant used to make the *umuthi* (medicine or potion) for annual protection rituals, which protect people, animals, and crops and the spaces they inhabit from witchcraft. Gogo was growing intelezi so that she could protect her home, her garden, and her family. While Gogo Ngcobo had a sophisticated understanding of nutrition and its importance for health, she also understood that she needed to protect herself and her family from witchcraft.

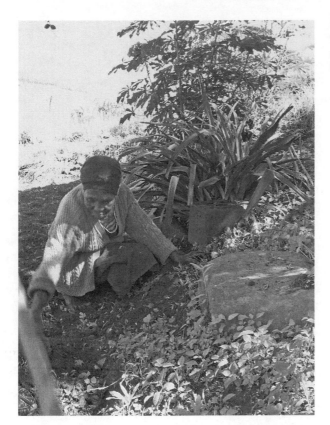

Figure I.2 Intelezi from Gogo Ngcobo's garden just behind her. Photo by author.

Gogo Ngcobo grew up in the catchment of a major social medicine program. In 1940, in a rare moment of concern for the health and welfare of all South Africans, the government sent a young, untested team to a remote, mountainous area in an African Reserve in what was then the province of Natal to set up the Pholela Community Health Centre (PCHC). Together, they developed an experiment in social medicine that became known as community-oriented primary care (COPC). This new brand of social medicine stressed the social as well as the biological causes of illness, blending clinical care at the health center with health education and extension work in the homes of area residents. This multisited approach required the efforts of doctors, nurses, health educators, *and* Pholela's residents, as the health center sought to improve health and lives collaboratively. And it did. Infant and crude mortality plummeted, gross malnutrition all but disappeared, and new cases of illnesses like syphilis decreased markedly. Just a decade after its inception, and by many measures, the PCHC was a rousing success. It was so effective, in fact, that it has been referred to as "a model for the world," and some call it one of the most successful social medicine interventions in history.[3]

As the conversations I had with Gogo Ngcobo in her garden reveal, the work of the PCHC shaped the ways in which residents understand their health and the homesteads they reside in. Gogo Ngcobo's comprehension of the role of food in health, her eating habits, her own good health, and the scientific form of her garden reveal the long-lasting impacts of the social medicine developed in Pholela. In many senses, Gogo Ngcobo and her garden offer a picture of the success of the health center's work in transforming homesteads and improving health. But Gogo's garden shows something else too. It shows that she continued to be concerned about illnesses the health center could not see or treat. The intelezi in the garden reveals that the health center's approach to healing was not monolithic. Gogo Ngcobo and her homestead inhabited two different, if interconnected, worlds of health and healing.

This book offers a story of social medicine, written from an out-of-the way place in sub-Saharan Africa that happens to be one of its most important origin sites. It tells a story of social medicine's possibilities and limitations through the lives, homesteads, and health of the people who were the subjects of the Pholela Community Health Center's experiment. As such, it offers an alternative to more common accounts, which tend to feature laudatory narratives of white, male doctors who practice medicine to fight for social justice. While doctors are an important part of this story, they are not at its center; Pholela's residents are. In this place, people lived in and made different worlds as they got sick and became well. These worlds were populated by people, things, and harder-to-categorize beings like ancestors. From the PCHC's perspective, there was one health reality on top of which different sets of "beliefs" accumulated. The way to understand and intervene in health outcomes was through scientific study, not through consultation with ancestors. Gogo Ngcobo's garden challenges this singularity. The worlds that residents and their gardens occupy shaped health outcomes in ways social medicine could not always understand and treat. For all of its many successes, the PCHC was limited by its own faith in science, both biomedical and social, as well as by broader political-economic forces at work in South Africa.

In the story I tell here, the successes and failures of social medicine resulted from the relationships among humans, nonhumans, and harder-to-categorize beings. Some of these relationships, like those between livelihoods and health, the PCHC recognized and actively worked to shift, drawing on the best social science of the time. But it did not and could not see all of the relationships.

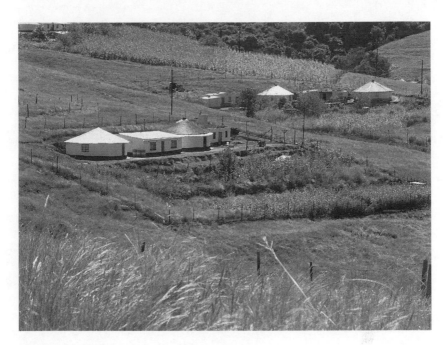

Figure I.3 Homesteads in Pholela. Photo by author.

For example, the PCHC failed to take account of Pholela's residents' roles in the development of its practice, and it never recognized the sociality of the nonhuman things (nutrients, protected water sources) that were integral to its program. Moreover, the PCHC did not understand how important Pholela-specific social relationships, including those with ancestors, were to health and healing. Paying attention to social medicine in Pholela reveals that unexpected and entangled more-than-human relationships are the basis of social life and health and healing. By starting with relationships, this book offers a vision of social life in which individual actors disappear and health and illness emerge as the product of entanglements.

To make this relational approach to health and healing clearer, I return to Gogo Ngcobo's garden. In some senses, the form of the garden, its diversity, and her ongoing good health could be attributed to the lessons she learned as a girl and the influence of the PCHC's health educators. It was also testament to the relationships she and her family developed with the PCHC and with the things of health center work, like seeds and nutrients. The limitations of COPC remained visible in the garden and in our conversations too. The garden was small; its contents could last only a couple of weeks after the last harvest. As a result, Gogo Ngcobo and her family bought most of the food they ate. Gogo's concern over processed maize meal reveals an anxiety about the ways in which racial capitalism curtailed the nutritional and health-related possibilities she and her family had access to by restricting land and wages for Africans. (Racial capitalism refers to the idea that capitalism has always been co-constituted with racism.)[4] Gogo's understanding of her limited food was evidence of the work of the PCHC and its health education efforts. While the health center could help residents modify homesteads and offer clinical care, it could not change the broad structures of racial capitalism that shaped livelihoods and health. This was not its only limit; the intelezi Gogo grew in her garden and her slight embarrassment at being asked about it (in the larger context of a conversation about agriculture and nutrition) reveal a second limit. This plant, the illness it was to prevent, and the world of health and healing it came from pose a challenge to an understanding of social life circumscribed by the social sciences. In Gogo Ngcobo's good health and her knowledge, and in her garden's contents and form, the relationships that set the stage for both the possibilities and the limitations of the PCHC's social medicine remain visible to this day.

The Story of Social Medicine, Commonly Told

Social medicine, the marriage of an attention to the social determinants of health with clinical care, has a long history, most often told from Europe and North America. A representative narrative of social medicine traces its roots to nineteenth-century Germany, where the scientist Rudolph Virchow called medicine a social science and combined an attention to pathology with statistical data collected at the population scale. The solutions to health problems that he proposed tended to be political, focused on broad-scale political changes like access to affordable housing, clean water, and education. These, he asserted, were the bases for health.[5] In this vision, the "social" of social medicine is couched in terms of what basic services the state could provide to its people. In 1920, the United Kingdom's government commissioned the Dawson Report, the blueprint for what would become the National Health Service. This report called for universally accessible medicine and is often credited as one of the foundational documents of social medicine.[6] Soon thereafter, in the 1930s in the United States, a medical historian named Henry Sigerist wrote about and advocated for what he called "socialized medicine." By socialized, he was referring to an attention to the factors that made some people sicker than others and a practice that addressed those factors.[7] He later helped to construct Canada's national health care program. Following these threads, in the middle of the twentieth century, Thomas McKeown used population-scale data to argue that late nineteenth-century population growth in England was due to improvements in economic conditions, public health, and access to medicine, rather than rises in fertility.[8] This analysis centered the very kinds of medical and social programs so crucial to social medicine.

The ideas of these men and these reports traveled around the world. In Latin America, social medicine became a rallying cry of revolutionaries like Argentine doctor Che Guevara in Cuba and President Salvador Allende in Chile. These leaders asserted that access to health care and the basic building blocks of a healthy life were key for functioning societies. As such, they used concerns over health to call for a comprehensive restructuring of society and a redistribution of wealth. For these leaders, economic status was the basis for health, as economics represented the social of social medicine. While not directly related, what happened in Pholela and South Africa more generally was part of this bigger story of social medicine. The typical story of the PCHC opens with the arrival of Sidney and Emily Kark, two young doctors of European descent, and their team in 1940 to set up the Pholela Community Health Center. In Pholela, they, along with additional doctors who came later, developed their own brand of social medicine (COPC) and then wrote about and taught it both in South Africa and in countries like Israel and the United States.[9] At about the same time that social medicine was catching on in Latin America and South Africa, the Chinese government developed its own form of social medicine through its barefoot doctors program. In this program the government trained peasants to travel around the countryside and treat common ailments, thereby extending medical care to the rural poor.[10] All of these social medicine efforts shifted the focus away from individual bodies to the societies in which people lived as political-economy and public health became the framework for understanding social life in health.

At the global scale, the rising interest in social medicine was part of a broader movement to improve the lives of the world's poor. It was also rooted in the growing idea that health is a human right, which was first articulated in the United Nations' 1948 Universal Declaration of Human Rights. In addition, the broader history is connected to an increasing recognition that the inequities that colonialism and imperialism wrought in places like Africa led to drastically different expectations and possibilities for people depending on where they lived and what race and gender they were. This focus on social medicine culminated in the 1978 Alma Ata Declaration on primary health care for all. Coauthored by Sidney Kark, this declaration asserted that all people in the world had the right to both a healthy life and the primary health care they would need to sustain that life.

This is a conventional story of social medicine and an important one. It offers some key people, policies, and documents, which lay the foundation for this invaluable branch of medicine, and it shows its global reach. But it is also a very white and a very male story. With the exception of China's program, all of the leaders I write about here were either European or of European descent, trained in universities in Europe or universities staffed by European- or American-trained professors. As a result, this story of social medicine is a new twist on an old story of universal science developed in the Global North and transported and applied around the world. Its focus on people living in poverty and on primary health care offers a slight alternative, but only a slight one. Much of the recent literature on global health follows similar patterns, focusing on formal programs run out of institutions in the Global North.[11] These programs are invested in the extension of biomedicine to people and places in the Global South. These are stories of Euro-American medicine in Africa and Latin America. The story most commonly told of Pholela is no different; the doctors take center stage as their work and ideas travel.[12] They are the face of social medicine, the face of the people living in poverty. This is not that story.

Pholela and South Africa in the 1930s

In the 1930s, Pholela, South Africa, was part of the African Reserve area of KwaZulu in the province of Natal. Nestled in the foothills of the southern Drakensberg Mountains, the district sits in a messy patchwork where communally held African land is mixed in among European (white) farms and small European-occupied towns. Though apartheid would not officially begin until 1948, there had long been policies and practices of dispossession of and discrimination against African populations, part of what Patrick Wolfe refers to as the apparatus of settler colonialism.[13] In the nineteenth and early twentieth centuries, economic and minority interests coalesced into policies that forced native Africans onto smaller and smaller pieces of land called Native Reserves, forcibly settling nomadic and seminomadic peoples like the ancestors of Pholela's residents. This dispossession meant that whites gained access to extensive parcels of land for agricultural production, mining and other natural resource extraction, and industry, which was key to making South Africa the biggest economy on the continent.

These policies first coalesced in the 1913 Natives Land Act, which made it illegal for Africans to own or lease land in white areas.[14] On the eve of the establishment of the PCHC, African Reserves made up 11.7 percent of the land in South Africa and housed the vast majority of Africans, who made up 69 per-

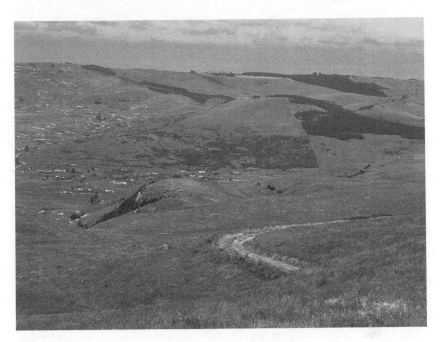

Figure I.4 A view of Pholela from a mountaintop. The lines between communally held African land and white-owned land are clear even now. Today most of the white-owned land remains in tree plantations rather than agriculture as it had been in the 1940s and 1950s. Photo by author.

cent of the country's population.[15] The gross inequities in land occupation meant that most rural Africans had only limited space for agriculture and few or no opportunities to expand their production. With less land to cultivate, limited pasture for livestock, soil erosion, and increasing administrative controls like the "hut" tax, which required men to pay an annual tax based on the number of buildings they had on their homestead, large numbers of African males entered into migrant labor, leaving their families behind because of laws requiring Africans to carry passes in white areas.[16]

Pholela exemplified this political reality. The doctors who established the PCHC often commented that one of the most striking features of the landscape was its lack of men, and in particular, young men. These young men sent remittances home from the nominal wages they earned for their low-skilled work, supporting their families from afar.[17] The family members who stayed behind worked what little land they had available, and they used remittances to buy processed maize meal and other staples (if they could afford them) to supplement their meager agricultural yields. The combined livelihood approach of women's agriculture at home and men's low-wage labor away meant that families barely survived and that their health often suffered. This was what racial capitalism looked like in Pholela.

When they returned home, the men brought new diseases like syphilis and tuberculosis with them, where they took root in their malnourished families and neighbors. As residents began to suffer from unfamiliar illnesses, they understood and treated them through a preexisting framework of health and healing. In Pholela, as in much of sub-Saharan Africa, illnesses are divided into three broad categories: illnesses from ancestors, illnesses from witchcraft, and illnesses that just happen, which was the most common category.[18] The most important difference came in etiology: an illness could "just happen" or it could be the product of intent, caused by a person like an angry ancestor or an *umthakathi* (a person who sends witchcraft). Determining the category of an illness was the key first step in alleviating symptoms and making a person well, because each type of illness had a different treatment regimen. For illnesses that just happen residents visited a nurse or a doctor; for witchcraft or ancestor illness they visited a healer who works with the ancestors (an *umthandazi* or an *isangoma*). But it was rarely clear what type of illness a person had.[19] As a result, Pholela's residents often tacked back and forth between biomedicine and various traditional healers. It was into this context that the PCHC entered in 1940. And it was this political, economic, and health context that would come to shape the possibilities and limitations of the social medicine that developed in this place.

Scholarly Threads

To understand social medicine from Pholela, I offer a political ecology of health approach.[20] With this approach, I understand health and healing as ontological and constitutive of worlds. By this I mean that I recognize that the physical manifestation of illness is as significant as its sociocultural relationships, and further that the two are entangled; I start from the position that the worlds we live in are relationally produced.[21] In other words, people, things, plants, animals, and harder-to-categorize beings like ancestors are what they are because of the relationships they are entangled in, relationships that are more than human. Furthermore, the worlds they inhabit and constitute are entangled and interconnected; they are the product of these relationships.[22] The understanding of health, healing, and worlds I offer here builds on the work of scholars interested in political ecology, ontology, medical anthropology, and science studies.

To set up a political-ecology analysis, I begin with an examination of how the PCHC's social medicine ordered and intervened in Pholela. To do this, I draw on medical anthropology and science studies scholarship, which reveal that supposedly universal sciences like biomedicine are socially and culturally local and produced through relationships.[23] This scholarship highlights the role of people like Gogo Ngcobo in the production of science and scientific knowledge, as she and her garden represent the social medicine that came from Pholela. But understanding Gogo's role is not enough for understanding social medicine from Pholela, where homestead transformation and things like vegetables and nutrients were integral to health center practice. For this, I draw on science studies scholars interested in questions of nonhuman agency. These scholars argue that science is the product of relationships among people and things, where things can act just as people can. One particularly valuable framework for this is the assemblage, which centers human–nonhuman relationships and articulates agency relationally.[24] This scholarship helps to make the PCHC's vision of practice clear, offering an examination of its remarkable success. Gogo's garden's contents and organization and her ongoing good health five decades after the PCHC lost its funding are testaments to the importance and success of human–nonhuman assemblages.

While science studies and medical anthropology help to critically interrogate social medicine as a science, political ecology, inflected by scholarship on racial capitalism, helps to illuminate some of the limits of the social medicine practiced in Pholela. Combining an attention to political economy (through the social sciences) and an attention to the biology of ecosystems and bodies (through ecology and biomedicine), political ecology reveals that the gardens and fields of Pholela's residents were inextricably linked to the health of the people, and moreover, that both were shaped by the broad political-economic processes at work in South Africa and Pholela.[25] This understanding of the importance of political economy also underpinned the PCHC's social medicine practice, where social life was understood through a Marxist analysis of South Africa's political economy and Pholela's livelihoods. Because the political economy of South Africa has always been stratified by race, work on racial capitalism is particularly valuable for a political-ecology analysis in this place. While most often traced to Cedric Robinson's foundational work, *Black Marxism: The Making of the Black Radical Tradition*, the term *racial capitalism* was first articulated by scholars working in and on South Africa.[26] These scholars understood that capitalism and more, capitalist accumulation, were predicated on a racial hierarchy enforced by both government policy and industrial practices. These policies and practices, which culminated in apartheid, ensured astonishing profits for whites at the expense of African laborers. This is a pattern that continues to this day, shaping the health and illness of South Africa's poorest people, as Mark Hunter has so aptly demonstrated in his work on the implications of a livelihood strategy that includes everyday sexual transactions for HIV rates.[27] Understanding social medicine and the work of the PCHC through a political ecology informed by racial capitalism reveals that notions of racial inferiority as well as questions of funding shaped the sciences that underpinned social medicine. It also reveals that no matter how innovative and progressive the PCHC's social medicine program was, it could not overcome the larger forces that circumscribed livelihoods and the possibilities for healthy futures for Africans in South Africa. Gogo Ngcobo certainly knew this as she discussed her anxieties about the insufficient harvest of her garden, the inferiority of processed food, and the impact both had on her health. She understood that her health was connected to the limited livelihood possibilities of her family through food.

Racial capitalism was not the only force to shape and limit social medicine in Pholela; the multiple worlds of health and healing of residents also determined what was possible. As my conversation with Gogo Ngcobo makes clear, for residents, nutrients and vegetables (and the relationships with the health center that they were a part of) were important for health. Likewise, as the intelezi in Gogo Ngcobo's garden reveals, relationships with neighbors and ancestors and the various components of traditional medicine were important to health. For the PCHC, witchcraft was not real; it was a product of belief and proof of a population not yet educated in scientific medicine. But in Pholela, people suffered and still continue to suffer from witchcraft illnesses that can only be treated with traditional medicine. The ongoing importance of traditional medicine reveals that the social relationships that the PCHC did not and could not recognize among neighbors and between the living and their ancestors were important to both health and healing. To understand a vision of social life embedded in witchcraft illnesses, I draw on anthropological literature on medical pluralism and health and healing in Africa. Medical pluralism recognizes that both biomedicine and traditional medicine are important and viable options for healing for many people around the world, and Africanist literature roots health and healing in African social worlds.[28] Together, these bodies of scholarship offer a framework of cultural specificity and social construction for incorporating witchcraft illnesses into an examination of social medicine.

But the articulation of different regimes of health and healing as sociocultural does not fully grapple with the physicality of illness.[29] For this, I draw on the work of feminist science studies scholars and scholars interested in questions of ontology. This scholarship focuses on the entanglements of the physicality of illness and sociocultural relationships. I find this scholarship particularly generative because of its focus on the irreducibility of (social) relationships to ontology and in this case to physical health.[30] In this thinking, there are no individuals or individual elements; things and people come into being through their relationships, which make up the human–nonhuman world. This approach to relationality is particularly generative for understanding health from Pholela because it decenters scientific ways of understanding and opens up the possibility that more-than-human actors like ancestors and witchcraft, actors that science does not recognize, can have an impact on bodily health. Take the example of the intelezi in Gogo Ngcobo's garden. Gogo grew this plant so that she could use it for an umuthi that an isangoma would make to protect her home and the people who lived in it from ill health and misfortune due to witchcraft. For the intelezi to work, the isangoma must enlist the help of Gogo's ancestors, who are key for maintaining health. For this thing (the intelezi) to prevent illness, it requires a number of humans, nonhumans, and harder-to-categorize beings.

With intelezi growing alongside vegetables like beetroot, Gogo Ngcobo's garden reveals that residents occupied more than one world of health and healing. To understand this multiplicity, I draw on the work of Stacey Langwick, who demonstrates that biomedicine and traditional medicine are not separate for the people who practice them. Instead, each helps the other by attending to the physical manifestations of illness and the different social relations that are integral to it.[31] Further, through efforts to heal and the therapeutic objects with which to do so, Langwick sees moments of "ontological coordination." These moments reveal how worlds of health and healing are made and remade for and by the people she works with.[32] For Pholela's residents like Gogo Ngcobo, ontologies are multiple, relational, and overlapping.[33] This multiplicity exposes another limit to the social medicine practiced in Pholela.

Taken together, this scholarship helps to probe the possibilities and limitations of social medicine, expand understandings of health to be always relational and more than human, and offers possibilities for a different, more expansive vision of social life and social medicine. In the age of global health, the social medicine that Pholela's residents and their homes suggest we need includes actors often glossed as cultural, like ancestors, and recognizes their role in illness and health for the people who are so often the targets of global health programs.[34] Understanding health as relational and including these actors offers not just a different story of social medicine, but the story of a different social medicine.[35] As Vandana Shiva writes, "Since creativity has diverse expressions, I see science as a pluralistic enterprise that refers to different 'ways of knowing.' For me, it is not restricted to modern Western science, but includes the knowledge systems of diverse cultures in different periods of history."[36] In this framework, social medicine from Pholela is a science, one that offers possibilities for global health.

Sources and Methods

My ethnographic practice focuses on the health-related practices and the lived experience of illness and healing for Pholela's residents. Since 2008, I have worked closely in and with three communities in Pholela, which I call Enkangala, Ethafeni, and Entabeni.[37] Key to the research design, Enkangala and Ethafeni sit in what was once the catchment of the PCHC, while Entabeni sits outside. This spatial division provides for an understanding of what changes might have been instigated by the health center and what were the result of other local and national forces. It also offers a pathway for understanding health outside of the influence of the PCHC. I have conducted the vast majority of my ethnographic research in these three communities with Thokozile Nguse, who has been at least equal parts sister, interlocutor, and research assistant.[38] While Thokozile and I got to know and spend time with many people in these places, most of our work involved eight households with whom we conducted detailed oral histories about health and livelihoods between 1955 and 2009. Our conversations, observations, and experiences with these people and others form the backbone of the research for this book. (Chapter 2 describes this research in detail.) My time in Pholela also shapes the form of the book, which tacks back and forth between past and present, much as our oral histories, interviews, and conversations did.

Of equal importance to the details and stories gathered through time spent in Pholela is the analytical value of ethnographic research. To understand this, I draw inspiration from Sarah Hunt's claim that stories are ontologies. By this, I mean that stories aren't metaphors; they don't need to be explained through comparison. Instead, they represent realities.[39] The best way to understand stories is therefore by getting to know the places and people from which they emerge. The informal conversations Thokozile and I participated in and the observations we have made over more than a decade provide much of the basis for my analysis of health, healing, and social medicine in Pholela. After all, thinking about social medicine *from* Pholela requires a firm grounding in the worlds—the ontologies—of area residents; ethnography offers one important way to access these worlds.

For a historical perspective, I analyzed archival documents from the PCHC, and its publications, and drew on regional ethnographies of Nguni-speaking peoples.[40] Rich in detail, these sources offer a wealth of information on the life and ideas of Africans, life at the moment of the establishment of the PCHC and after, health center practices, and residents' engagement in the work of the health center. In particular, PCHC publications offer valuable data and analyses of household surveys and experiences in Pholela and important insight into the views and work of the health center's doctors. These sources are not without their own biases and problems, however, which is part of the reason that they are so helpful for understanding the PCHC's vision of social medicine, which I examine in chapter 1.

A third group of sources includes scientific papers on nutrition and health.[41] This work helped me examine the role of, for example, nutrients in health, or the specific nature of kwashiorkor, an illness caused by an acute protein deficiency. As such, they help explain the "matter" of social medicine (at least in the world of health and healing where biomedicine is at work), just as government reports and publications help to explain its "meaning."[42] These are key documents for the political-ecology approach at work in chapter 3. When coupled with oral sources and ethnographies, which offer insight into the meaning and matter of witchcraft diseases (the subject of chapter 4), these scientific sources help provide a rich picture of health in Pholela.

Given the diversity of written and other sources, reading and integrating these various pieces of research is both particularly important and particularly challenging. To do so, I offer a method of entanglement and diffraction. Building on Donna Haraway's and Karen Barad's concept of diffraction, I read and incorporate sources through one another, attending to their "interaction, interference, reinforcement, [and] difference."[43] In particular, diffraction offers a way to attend to difference and change over time and across space, as well as a way to examine spaces of overlap. Moreover, as Barad writes, diffraction "is not just a matter of interference, but of entanglement."[44] In other words, attending to difference is not enough; one must attend to the coproduction that occurs as a result of the intra-actions of different sources. Here, I use the term *intra-action* (as opposed to interaction), putting to work Barad's idea that all beings are relational from the start; this is especially valuable for understanding coproduction.[45] A key insight of the concept of diffraction is that the researcher plays an integral role in research produced.[46] Recognizing this, of course, means that I must acknowledge that the analysis offered in this book is diffracted through my experience and knowledge (as well as through my relationships, experiences, and conversations with Thokozile), through the lives and words of Pholela's residents, the writings of the PCHC's staff, and scientific understandings of nutrients and bacteria. This book is a result of these entanglements.[47]

What emerges is not a neat and tidy story; it is a story of interconnected worlds, worlds in which social medicine is many things simultaneously and social life is broad, relational, and more than human. Through a method of diffraction, seemingly contradictory sources intra-act and offer new possibilities and new insights. Consider the example of physical illness. Reading symptoms through its manifestation in the body, the diagnosis of a doctor, the work of an isangoma, the explanation of an ill person, and my own ideas and experience offer a somewhat contradictory but rich view of illness, wellness, social life, and the worlds of health and healing in Pholela. This method of diffraction, attuned to difference, opens up the possibility that health and social medicine are even more complex than what well-known histories offer and the staff of the PCHC imagined.

1

Seeing Like
a Health Center

A fresh-faced twenty-nine-year-old medical doctor arrived in the Pholela region of the KwaZulu Bantustan in January of 1940. Dr. Sidney Kark had graduated from the University of the Witwatersrand's Medical School just four years earlier.[1] In the intervening time, he had worked as a medical doctor in African Reserves and as a social scientist conducting epidemiological research.[2] He arrived in Pholela with a small interracial team, which included his wife, Emily, a doctor; Edward and Amelia Jali, a Zulu health aide and a trained nurse; and a couple of Zulu-speaking health educators.[3] The government sent this young, capable, and energetic team to set up the country's first rural health center.[4] The team hoped that their work in Pholela would prove that the best way to enhance overall health was through a program of health education, clinical care, and social support at the community scale.

By 1952, just twelve years after the government had established the PCHC, the team's careful epidemiological analysis showed its efforts to be remarkably successful. In the clinic's target population, infant mortality had dropped by 64.8 percent, crude mortality (the overall death rate) had fallen from 38.3 percent in 1942 to 13.6 percent in 1950, syphilis infection rates were lower, malnutrition had decreased tenfold, and periodic epidemics of typhoid and scabies had all but disappeared.[5] The social medicine the health center had pioneered was nothing short of remarkable. And yet its success merits investigation. In this chapter, I probe why the PCHC was so successful, how that success was articulated, and what that success teaches about the way the health center understood health, and in particular the role of social life in health. Doing so helps to uncover the possibilities and limitations of social medicine.

In order to prove its success, the PCHC had to measure it, and statistics became a way to do so. After all, making its success legible was crucial for maintaining support, and measurement was a precursor for legibility. James Scott famously demonstrated that making landscapes and populations legible through a process of naming, cataloging, measuring, codifying, and mapping was fundamental to the production of the modern state. These efforts, Scott argues, allowed the state, via various development schemes, to see and govern new populations and places through the application of scientific knowledge and technocratic approaches.[6] In order to measure its success, the PCHC did something similar. It had to construct Pholela's communities as measurable units. This meant that the PCHC needed to make the household and the community meaningful scales of analysis. In defining these scales, the health center staff used ideas based in the social sciences about what constitutes a family and a community as well as social science methods that fixed these scales through data collection. In so doing, the PCHC mapped a particular vision of social life onto Pholela. To be sure, Pholela already contained communities, as well as separate households, that were largely tied to individual families. But the work the PCHC did to improve health, to study homesteads and communities, and to render their practice legible to the outside world offered new meanings to these scales, hardened existing boundaries, and created new ones.

Once the PCHC clearly articulated the scales of the homestead and the community, it developed a practice through which to address the health of the individual, family, and community simultaneously, all with an attention to the national political economy. This multiscalar practice sought to intervene in the social world of Pholela's residents and the biology of landscapes and bodies to enhance community health by improving the health of families and individuals. Seeing like a health center means seeing through biological and social science lenses and understanding and enacting a practice that links individuals and their health to the nation through their homesteads and communities. But as the example of a typhoid outbreak reveals, in practice, the PCHC could see past its vision of social life, prizing improvements in health and recognizing that reality was complex.

The Roots of the Pholela Community Health Centre

Welfare for All? National Development Schemes in the 1930s and 1940s

When the health center team arrived in Pholela in 1940, they were backed by a national government that was interested in improving the lives of its entire population. In the 1930s and 1940s, interest in the health and welfare of the country's African population reached the highest levels of government. This led to the production of a number of research reports on Africans as well as organizations and institutions dedicated to promoting their health and welfare.[7] This ethos made the establishment of the PCHC possible, while lending official support to the experiment in social medicine that would be carried out.

South Africa was not alone in working to address the needs of the people in greatest economic distress. In the wake of World War I and the Great Depression, a number of countries around the world expanded their social welfare programs, and colonial powers grew increasingly interested in "development" initiatives.[8] In South Africa, this meant extending old age and disability pensions to nonwhite people, as well as the development and expansion of progressive policies and institutions. It also meant taking the information collected on household composition, nutrition, and economics to create a series of policies and programs to promote the health and welfare of all South Africans through the application of scientific best practices.[9] It was during this moment that the South African government began its experiment in community health, first establishing the PCHC and then the National Health Services Commission under soon-to-be Minister of Health Harry Gluckman (brother of the renowned anthropologist Max Gluckman). This commission was charged with better understanding and addressing the health needs of the African population. Out of this came the health center model, which began in Pholela and was replicated in more than fifty sites around the country in the 1940s and 1950s. This and other programs developed in this progressive moment shared a common belief in the power of data-driven policy developed through the application of social science methods, the promise of scientific intervention, and an ethos of self-help, whereby Africans living in poverty, with the help of government agents, would engage in various scientifically informed practices to "help themselves."

South African history is often seen as a smooth and inevitable march from the colonial period to minority rule and then to apartheid, which began officially in 1948 and became more draconian (what is known as high apartheid) at the end of the 1950s. But the interwar period complicates that narrative. The expansion of government programs and presence in places like Pholela in the 1930s and 1940s was based on the radical premise that everyone, regardless of race, had the right to a healthy and productive life. In the short time before apartheid, members of the South African government as well as scholars were working toward a slightly different South Africa than the one in which they were living. This South Africa extended (limited) social welfare benefits to all people, and it created new development schemes in places long ignored by the state. At the same time, it left segregation unchallenged. This was the context in which the Karks were trained and in which the government established the Pholela Community Health Centre in 1940.

The Making of Social Medicine Practitioners

When the Karks arrived in Pholela,[10] they came with several ideas about how to practice community medicine. These ideas had taken root a decade earlier when they were students at the prestigious English-language University of the Witwatersrand (Wits) in Johannesburg. In 1929, eighteen-year-old Sidney Kark entered the medical school at Wits and soon met Emily, who was also a medical student. At the university, they had a typical biomedical education, where they learned about health in individual bodies.[11] After classes and years of clinical training, they graduated as highly trained doctors who rivaled new physicians from the Global North. During their hands-on training, they had opportunities to visit parts of South Africa they had never seen before, witnessing the lives of the majority of the country's African population for the first time. These experiences helped lay the foundation for the work they would do in Pholela.

But their training was not simply about pathology and physiology. The Karks also took classes in the social sciences and humanities taught by a number of well-known, progressive faculty members. In these classes, they learned about Marxist interpretations of South Africa's class structure and political economy, what the Karks later called "socio-economic historical analysis."[12] They learned about the problems created by the country's racial divides and the realities of life for the majority of South Africa's poor Africans. They learned that the difficult lives and ill health of many Africans could be attributed to a long history of oppression, disenfranchisement, and race-based economic inequality, what is today called racial capitalism.[13] The Karks also learned how to conduct social science research. For example, Professor Winifred Hoernlé, who founded the program in social anthropology at Wits, taught the Karks about social science methods, particularly long-term fieldwork. Studying with her had an important influence on the (qualitative) methods the Karks would use in COPC, especially their reliance on participant observation.

The professors at Wits taught that improving the lives of South Africans living in poverty could only happen by addressing systemic issues: oppression, disenfranchisement, and economic inequality at national and local scales. When applied to health, this approach addressed what is now referred to as the social determinants of health, recognizing the role of racial capitalism in setting the terms of what is possible. Eustace Cluver, for example, lectured on public health and focused on the neglect of African people in both public health and medical interventions. By implication, he taught that the first step to improving health was to offer health care to Africans. Lessons like these were crucial for the Karks as they came to imagine life as medical practitioners serving South Africa's poor African population.

The professors at Wits also pushed their students to act, insisting that they had a responsibility to do so. To that end, some of their professors introduced the Karks to the nascent South African Institute of Race Relations (SAIRR). The SAIRR is an organization dedicated to research and awareness about racial inequality in South Africa and the political struggle to end segregation and oppression.[14] It provided the Karks with a model for a marriage between research and theory on the one hand, and political action on the other. For the Karks, who were active in progressive student politics, this was particularly valuable and helped guide their work in Pholela and beyond.[15] The ideas they encountered in classrooms and from the SAIRR were radical in a country with a long history of racist ideology codified into law. These experiences transformed the Karks from medical students occupied with anatomy, pathology, and other components of a biomedical education, to future physicians dedicated to social change and concerned with the broad social and cultural factors that shape both health and health care delivery.

Immediately after his medical training, Sidney took a position with the Ministry of Health to conduct a large-scale survey of the nutrition of African schoolchildren throughout South Africa. He worked on a team with Edward Jali, the university-trained health aide who would join him in Pholela. The survey offered Kark and Jali hands-on training in social science survey methods and analysis, provided them with the opportunity to visit new parts of the country, and gave them the time and space to develop a relationship. What they found through their work was both surprising and disheartening: 70 percent of African boys and 66 percent of girls surveyed suffered from some degree of malnutrition.[16] This confirmed what Kark had learned at Wits: malnutrition was a systemic rather than an individual problem, and it affected Africans living in poverty the most. Kark's work on the Bantu Nutrition Survey had a deep impact on the way he understood the importance of nutrition for health and the value of comprehensive surveys for social medicine. Indeed, this experience with social science research, like his training in South Africa's hospitals and clinics, would prove invaluable as he, Emily, Edward and Amelia Jali, and their team began their work developing COPC in Pholela.

Mapping the Community and the Household

From the start, the health center team's aim was to improve overall health in Pholela. Because of the broad nature of this goal, they needed a way to focus the intervention. They chose to concentrate on improving health at the community scale by targeting households. An important first step in developing a health center practice was therefore to define and delimit a community for intensive study and intervention; it was to make the community scale meaningful. To do this, the PCHC needed to decide what constituted a community. In other words, it needed to bound communities out of the people and landscapes of Pholela and make them legible to both residents and the outside world.[17]

As the health center began its health extension work, it set out to find its first community. To do this, the PCHC designated an area of roughly 130 households overlooking the Umkomaas River that it imagined to be a distinct community. For the PCHC, homesteads and the people who lived in them (households) were the basic building blocks of communities. The health center called this group of households the River View Area, what I refer to as Enkangala.[18] Enkangala mainly consisted of separate homesteads made up of a couple of round buildings with thatched, conical roofs, arranged on patches of bare red ground cut out of the otherwise grassy hillside. Clustered on the mountain slopes, divided from other similar clusters by rivers, forests, and ridgelines, these homesteads gave the appearance of a discrete community.

In some senses, this was correct. Clusters of homesteads like Enkangala were geographically contiguous; they usually represented an extended kinship network; and they often fell under a single headman (a political designation just below chief), making them distinct political units. Therefore, rather than a straightforward example of a development initiative defining a community for its own purposes, as Arun Agrawal and Clark Gibson describe in their work on community-based conservation, the PCHC's efforts to define communities were drawn from life in Pholela.[19] Indeed, without realizing it, the health center used the preexisting divisions of long-standing political hierarchies to determine the communities that would come to make up the Designated Area and that would be so important to health center practice.

Community was just one way of organizing and circumscribing health center work. One could imagine another program focused on a type of disease, or age (children or the elderly), or gender. If any of these factors had been the organizing feature of COPC, staff would have set out looking for anyone with tuberculosis or anyone over sixty, regardless of where she or he lived. Health assistants would then create maps that extended beyond a specific area but missed some of what was in the area. In these maps, physical features like roads and forests would become less important, while certain social or demographic characteristics would become more important. The spatial logic the health center used and the communities it imagined were not inherent to social medicine or to Pholela; they were the health center's vision. This vision, mapped through cartographic space and then enacted through specific programs, brought new meanings to preexisting communities, strengthened divisions among them, and made the scale itself meaningful. The maps would also make communities legible to the government and other funders and professionals, thereby helping people near and far get to know Pholela and support the PCHC.[20]

Health center efforts also changed the relationships between this place, its people and communities, and the state. In so doing, this process made communities different than they had been before the health center came to Pholela. In charting shifting meanings of the term *community* in African studies, Jane Guyer writes that scholarship over the past forty years has focused on community as "a local social structure and tradition of life within a wider stratified political and economic system under a state form of government."[21] Likewise, Agrawal and Gibson see *community* not as a taken-for-granted term for a small spatial unit, but as first and foremost a political term used by governments and other organizations.[22] This was clearly the case in the River View Area, which the PCHC designated and which was the only community in Pholela with an English name.[23]

Once they had chosen a community for the Designated Area, the health center staff began to collect data. Central to this process was defining the household.[24] The health center saw the household as the scale at which the most local landscape (the homestead) and the family came together. As a result, it would be the central site for the implementation of health center practice. Therefore, as the health center set out to collect data on the community, it did so through a *household* survey to augment its community mapping project. Guyer notes the importance of the household as a unit for research, arguing that its continued use in African studies scholarship has more to do with its methodological usefulness than with its meaning for Africans. In particular, she and others point out that it continues to hold power because it serves as a key economic unit.[25]

In Pholela, this was certainly the case. The household was the site where livelihood practices came together. In addition, for both the PCHC and the government more broadly, the household represented the family located in a specific place. In 1878, this particular vision of the homestead was codified into Native Law.[26] This now-legal definition of a homestead was an easy unit for

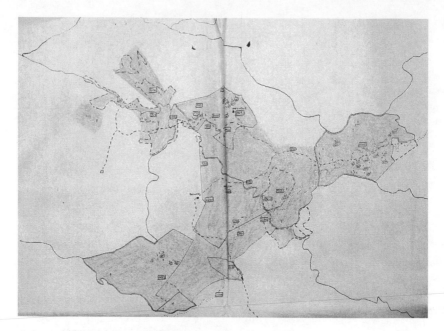

Figure 1.1 A map of the Designated Area with key landmarks, roads, and numbers of households. SAB, GES vol. 1917, ref. 46/32.

survey and census purposes. As a result, it became the key unit for social science research in South Africa. But, like the community, the household consists of a number of social relationships. As Guyer writes, the household refers to "a group constituted according to concepts, rights, obligations, and areas of freedom about marriage, parenthood, residence, work, and the constraints of making a living."[27] One important implication of this idea is that a household is not the stable unit so often presupposed in surveys. It evolves over time; it can be spatially diffuse (and was in Pholela); and it both shapes and is shaped by the political economy of the places in which it is located.

In fixing and defining households through its research efforts, the PCHC tried to account for their complexity, noting labor migration, local mobility among household members (especially kids), shifting homestead sites, and the presence of people who were not related to the family. The PCHC's understanding of the household anticipated many of the critiques scholars would offer forty years later. But its focus on the household as primarily an economic unit conforms to the understandings these scholars critique. It also reveals an understanding of social life focused on political economy. Because of the ways migrant labor underpinned racial capitalism in South Africa, understanding the household as an economic unit meant recognizing that it exceeded the spatial boundaries of the homestead. The health center certainly understood this. And yet, due to its focus on mapping and the practicalities of survey research, the health center fixed households in cartographic space, giving staff, government officials, and potential funders a sense of permanence that papered over a complicated reality.

Quantitative Social Science and the Household Survey

Just two years after the Karks and their team arrived in Pholela, the PCHC's five health assistants went into the newly demarcated Designated Area armed with the initial maps to conduct the first household survey. As they went door to door, they numbered homesteads, updated the original maps, and collected information on basic family demographics. They also paid careful attention to the immediate physical environment in which people lived, cataloging the number, type, size, and use of buildings, type of ventilation, general cleanliness, and waste disposal practices. In addition, health assistants collected information on agriculture, including garden and field yields, crop diversity, and livestock counts to better understand a family's food production and the contribution of home production to household livelihood strategies and nutrition-related health. Finally, to acquire a broad understanding of the health challenges facing Pholela, health assistants gathered data on the health history of individuals in each family. It recorded the information for each household in family files and then aggregated the data to get a blueprint of the community as a whole. Through this process, a picture of each household as the product of its people and the homestead environment emerged alongside an impression of a community consisting of several households.

The PCHC designed its data collection methods with an understanding that consistency and the ability to replicate data were preconditions for quality quantitative social science research. Sidney Kark and Edward Jali trained the health assistants who conducted the survey to ensure that it was carried out systematically with the most up-to-date methods. The health assistants documented everything they observed and they kept uniform records with the same information for each household. This practice helped to ensure that each piece of data was equivalent to the next, rendering each household equivalent to the next. This was high-quality social science research in action.

As time went on, the health center added new communities to its Designated Area, gathering more data and incorporating more households into its practice. Once collected on a community-by-community basis, the health cen-

TABLE D. (i)

NUMBER OF GARDENS WITH PARTICULAR VEGETABLE

IN JANUARY 1944.

Types of Vegetables arranged in rough order of frequency as at January 1944.	A 139 Homes surveyed		B 292 Homes surveyed		C. 261 Homes surveyed	
	No. of Homes with particular Veg.	% Incidence	No. of Homes with particular Veg.	% Incidence	No. of Homes with particular Veg.	% Incidence
Pumpkin	119	85.61	230	78.75	164	62.84
Potato	118	84.89	226	77.39	150	57.48
Bean	89	64.03	87	29.80	37	14.18
Cabbage	70	50.36	99	33.90	34	13.03
Tomato	59	43.44	105	35.96	10	3.83
Chinese Cabbage	53	38.14	91	31.16	28	10.73
Soyabean	52	37.15	96	32.88	1	0.38
Carrots	35	25.19	44	15.07	3	1.15
Sweetpotato	32	23.02	31	10.62	7	2.68
Pepper	29	20.86	41	14.04	17	6.51
Beetroot	26	18.71	33	11.30	0	0
Lucerne	25	17.99	43	14.72	0	0
New Zealand Spinach	24	17.27	26	8.90	6	2.30
Turnips	24	17.27	28	9.59	3	1.15
Peas	17	12.23	12	4.02	3	1.15
Shallott	16	11.51	52	17.80	15	5.75
"Amadumbi" (Taro)	12	8.63	12	4.02	8	3.06
Lettuce.	7	5.04	44	15.07	0	0

Other vegetables planted were "Ntshungu" (a local vine of which the leaves are eaten) - A7, B 18, C 10. "Imfe" (Sweet Cane) A 5, B 4, C 3. "Bece" (melon species) - A 5, B 6, C 5. Onions - A 5, B 17, C 1. Chou Mollier - A 3, B 9, C 0. Spinach Beet - A 2, B 0, C 0. Egg plant - A 2, B 0, C 0. Groundnut (Peanut) - A 2, B 2, C 3. Parsnip - A 1, B 0, C 0. Cucumber - A 1, B 1, C 0. Cauliflower - A 1, B 5, C 0. Groundbean ("Ndlubu Bean") - A 0, B 1, C 1.

(ii) NO. OF HOMES SURVEYED WHICH HAD NO VEGETABLE GARDENS IN JANUARY 1944.

Area A.	10	7.19%
Area B.	38	13.01%
Area C.	76	29.12%

Figure 1.2 An example of the results of the PCHC's garden survey from the 1944 Annual Report. SAB, GES vol. 1917, ref. 46/32.

ter totaled the data, offering a picture of health, agriculture, livelihoods, and homestead layout for the entire Designated Area, which it took to stand for all of Pholela. From these data, the health center came to determine that the average household had two fields, a small vegetable garden, and maybe one cow for food production. It found that the average homestead had a couple of buildings and no waste disposal system, and that four out of five men were away working in cities or on farms. In addition, these surveys confirmed what the health center staff had found in the clinic: the health picture in Pholela was bleak. Crude mortality rates were almost double the national average, there was gross mal-nutrition in 80 percent of the population, and there were higher than average rates of syphilis. Taken in aggregate and analyzed statistically, this information provided a baseline for community health against which extension efforts in the Designated Area would be measured.[28] The survey data also made Pholela's communities legible in a way that complemented the maps the health center produced, as statistics gave maps meaning.

To track its program and calculate its success, the PCHC needed not only to collect data annually, but to find a control group to measure its progress against. It did so through the case-control method of the social science of epidemiology. Every year between 1942 and the mid-1950s, the PCHC extended its Designated Area, incorporating new communities.[29] The so-called stepwise expansion always began with the production of a map and an initial household survey through which the health center delineated the boundaries of the community while also getting a baseline snapshot of its people, households, livelihoods, and health. In their first year, each new community became the "control" against which staff measured interventions. By comparing the communities already in the Designated Area to newly incorporated communities, the health center created something like a controlled experiment, the gold standard in scientific research. In theory, because these new communities were proximate to the pre-existing Designated Area, they were culturally the same and experienced the same outside forces. These similarities allowed the health center to control for influences other than its program when evaluating the efficacy of its practice.[30] Through this method, the community became a standard unit, much like the household and the individual, as each community was equivalent to the next thanks to the health center's consistent research program and its case-control method. This approach also helped to establish the community as a scale that was integral to the health center's methodology. But as the scholarship on community reveals, the assertion that each community was equivalent to the next was a fiction created to enable the kind of quantitative analysis that epidemiology requires.

A number of scholars have written about the tendency of science to take the "unruly complexity" of the human and natural worlds and make it neat and orderly through the process of categorization, data collection, and analysis.[31] This process is the hallmark of modern science and the modern state.[32] As Scott demonstrates, the production of scientific knowledge through the application of particular technologies like mapping and surveying is fundamental to the construction of the state. He argues that the modern state is built on a foundation of standardized and replicable data.[33] In many ways, the PCHC's use of research and data to define the community (and the household) are examples of what Scott writes about, especially insofar as the PCHC was part of a government project to improve the lives of Africans. After all, the production of data in Pholela required simplifying the place, its people, and the sociocultural relationships within it in order to develop a (biomedical and social) scientific practice.[34] For the PCHC, simplification was a prerequisite for the application of science.

Making this place and the social medicine practiced in it legible to the government, medical professionals, potential funders, and academics was at the heart of the mapping and surveying program. Defining the household and the community was central to that. Scholars studying global health have taken a renewed interest in how social science research, especially epidemiology, shapes how practitioners, governments, and funders understand places, projects, and people, and how they shape them.[35] In their work on AIDS research in Malawi, Crystal Biruk builds on Scott's argument to demonstrate that research and the production of data, especially quantitative survey data, is a sociocultural process that works to simplify reality to fit research priorities. This, Biruk argues, is a key precondition for understanding a problem (AIDS in this case) in order to intervene in and affect it. They write, "Underlying the ability of research projects to see the AIDS epidemic and to measure its effects on a population is the transformation of complexity into simplicity. Stories become marks in a survey box, people become data points, and households become dots on a map."[36] All of these processes were at work in Pholela: mapping, surveying, and defining (households, communities) were all preconditions for the establishment, the work and continuation, and the success of COPC. As Biruk demonstrates, this research has important effects as the stories these data tell about health, social life, and livelihoods are used to access resources and prove success.[37]

In Pholela, the survey work and epidemiological analysis that the health center conducted painted a picture of tremendous success. Aggregated for the entire Designated Area, the PCHC used these data to prove things like the 64.8 percent drop in infant mortality I note above or the 24 percent increase in households with home vegetable gardens that I write about in chapter 3. Statistics like these pepper this book, providing evidence for many of the claims I make. Indeed, it was because of these data that I went to Pholela in the first place. Even if statistics are limited in what they can see and how they represent reality, these numbers tell an impressive story, but a single story nonetheless. For the PCHC, this success meant funding from the Rockefeller Foundation after the apartheid government began to withdraw its financial support in the 1950s. But as Nolwazi Mkhwanazi reminds us in the context of global health programs today, there is a danger to a single story, especially a single story about health care in Africa.[38] It risks limiting understandings of health and social life to those defined by the health center.

The work of the PCHC in the 1940s and 1950s, with its focus on metrics and accounting, is reminiscent of the global health programs of today. Critical scholars of global health note that the focus on quantitative data collection and technological fixes like number of drugs delivered and number of patients diagnosed makes it difficult to attend to the heterogeneous on-the-ground reality that marks health and healing in places like Pholela.[39] This work includes, as Jane Guyer and colleagues write, the invention of numbers that underlie research and design.[40] This focus on the work of standardization and the possibilities and limitations of quantitative data is important for understanding the PCHC's vision of social medicine in Pholela, one that was rooted in and justified through numbers. As an early example of this kind of health intervention, the PCHC reveals the long history of a reliance on statistics in a health program.

The process by which the health center collected and analyzed its survey data ensured that the community and the family would be essential to the work of the PCHC in terms of both tracking progress and implementing programs. The quantitative social science implemented made the efficacy of health center work clear, helping to secure future funding, which ensured that the work would continue. It also helped to make COPC a brand of social medicine that governments and organizations would want to use. These research efforts reveal that the PCHC understood social life in terms of stable, definable units where relationships were predictable and the progression from smaller to larger (household to community) was straightforward.

Qualitative Social Science and the Family File

Drawing on their course work in anthropology, the Karks and their team developed the family file, in which they recorded information about each household and the individuals that made it up. The open-ended format allowed for discursive notes that did not fit in the strict form of the surveys. Each file contained information on the various people in the household, their school and work, and their health, as well as information about the homestead. These notes connected work in the clinic to work in the homestead, helping the nurses and doctors at the health center to make treatment plans that recognized individuals as members of a household. From the information in the files, they also produced narrative case studies, which told stories of individuals and families and how their health related to various aspects of social life, particularly political economy. This form of analysis allowed health center staff to grapple with the messy reality of life in Pholela that the surveys and maps obscured.

On a basic level, the family files affected how all residents of the Designated Area interacted with the health center. As residents recall, when they visited the PCHC, they told the receptionist their house number (RV 77, for example), and she or he pulled the family file for the doctor.[41] By the time a person was called into the examination room, the doctor and nurse had reviewed the file and had an understanding of the family situation. Reading about a brother who worked in Durban, a child who had died of measles, or a garden that yielded no beans (and therefore no protein), the doctor came to understand the social and ecological contexts in which the patient lived and experienced health. Likewise, when a patient visited the health center, the doctors recorded information in patient and family files that they thought important for understanding the different stresses—cellular, environmental, personal, social, and cultural—that might affect an individual's health. By diagnosing illness in the context of the family as a whole, the doctor presupposed a treatment plan that would likely involve the family, thereby linking the individual to the family in another way, through therapeutics. Through this practice, the health center inscribed new meaning to the family and to health care.

The notes from one particular family file from the annex of the 1944 Annual Report reveal how family files worked in practice. These notes describe a family and its trials with syphilis.[42] The health center's write-up of this case centers on the return of the head of the household. When this man got home, he went to the health center to get tested for syphilis. His test came back negative. Suspecting that his wife had been unfaithful while he was away working in Johannesburg, and knowing about the health center's system of recording information in a family file, he asked if it was safe for him to sleep with his wife. The health center understood that this man was using a health concern to gather information about his third wife's presumed infidelity. As the Karks write, "Fortunately for her she had attended [the health center] regularly for the previous seven months, and the Medical Officer was able to inform [her husband] that there was no danger."[43] Medically speaking, because this woman had received treatment for syphilis, she was not infected and the medical officer could tell the husband that he was not at risk for contracting the disease from his wife.

Practically and socially speaking, knowing the specifics of this family, and particularly the health center's detailed knowledge of this woman's sexual history, meant that the doctor understood that the husband was fishing for information about his wife's transgressions, rather than simply looking for information about a bacterial infection. The health center believed that the doctor's answer, which responded narrowly to the question of syphilis, would protect this woman from any retribution she might face for her infidelity, while delivering the medical advice the husband asked for. They credited their familiarity with the individuals in the family, thanks to homestead visits and the family file, with protecting this woman. They believed that this would preserve the family, which was taken as an unquestioned good. In this example, the health center's treatment of the woman as part of the family included not only antibiotics for the bacterium *Treponema pallidum*, but also careful management of familial relationships. In other words, treatment involved the bacteria, the individual, and the family.

Medical anthropologist Byron Good argues that the hierarchy embedded in the medical profession is an extension of the assumed "natural" hierarchy of the body in which cells make up organs, which make up the body.[44] In other words, he argues that in medicine, the body has its own scalar hierarchy. Geographers have long been interested in the production of spatial scales, recognizing them as the outcome of social relationships and political negotiations.[45] As Sallie Marston writes, "Scale is not necessarily a preordained hierarchical framework for ordering the world—local, regional, national and global. It is instead a contingent outcome of the tensions that exist between structural forces and the practices of human agents."[46] For the practitioners of social medicine who worked at the PCHC, their approach represented the marriage of the sociopolitical construction of the household–community scales with the cellular–body scales of biomedicine.[47] As this family file reveals, the nested hierarchy of the scales the health center worked with represented the blending of biomedicine with social science, as people and their health were located in a broader, legible and predictable, set of social relationships. For the PCHC, the family, especially in its connection to the household, was the key scale for linking the body to the community and the nation. But individuals and their families resist generalization, especially when it comes to the treatment plans of social medicine. As a result, the health center augmented their survey work with qualitative social science.

The Karks' training, especially in social anthropology, also comes through in the way they make sense of this case study. In this example, the unfaithful woman was the third wife of the head of the household. In their write-up, the doctors show no discomfort with polygamy, only with infidelity (defined as extramarital intimate relationships). And this appears to have less to do with a sense of morality than with the health center's focus on the household in its practice. To preserve the family, and by extension their practice, the doctors recognized that they needed to take the family on its own terms; in this instance, this meant accepting polygamy. For the Karks, the family was the preeminent social relationship, and it was defined by formal marriage ties. As the quote above continues: "Without the knowledge the Unit had regarding her adultery and his absence from home for lengthy periods, we might have been responsible for further undermining the stability of this family as well as the others involved."[48] As they saw it, the family was already on shaky ground thanks to a national economy dependent on migrant labor. Preserving the family was therefore a practical necessity and took a good deal of work and care. The family file, with its detailed information and attention to cultural norms and the larger political-economic context, made it possible for the health center to do that work.

This concern about keeping the family intact was an economic concern. Because the health center saw the household as the most important economic unit, it understood it to be the site where the social relations that political economy shaped affected individual health. The health center staff ends its write-up of this case study with three "social factors" that it blamed for "the immoral conduct" that led to the outbreak of syphilis throughout Pholela and in this household in particular: the necessity of male labor migration for household livelihoods, the lack of a sex life for a "virile young woman," and the repercussions of migration and libido on family life. In this accounting, the PCHC located the cause of syphilis in South Africa's political economy. Focusing on labor migration, Kark displaced responsibility for illness from the woman and her infidelity to the mandates of industrial and racial capitalism. As this case study makes clear, the health center saw political economy, not cultural practices like polygamy, as the most important social factor affecting health.[49]

The fact that the health center articulated its vision of the health of the individual as connected to the national political economy through a story is no accident. While scholars agree that poverty is bad for health, it is hard to trace the exact causal pathways that lead from inequality to diseases like syphilis. This story alone is about labor migration, government-mandated racial segregation, South Africa's industrial economy, gender relationships, household livelihood patterns, family formations, intimate encounters, and bacteria. These come together in a story because they all have a bearing on the health of this family, even though it is not perfectly clear how they come together and how each affects the other. This messiness is key for understanding the role of political economy as social life in health. The story in the case study, told from the collection of qualitative data, allows for this complexity in a way that the statistics of the household survey do not. As such, it reveals that the health center recognized the limits of what the quantitative social sciences could perceive and was willing to see beyond them. Seeing like a health center means seeing through stories as well as through surveys.

Developing a Health Center Practice:
Tracking, Mapping, and Controlling Outbreaks

Once the health center defined and studied people, households, and communities, it had to move on to implementing its social medicine practice. From its earliest days, the PCHC worked to control disease outbreaks like typhoid and scabies throughout Pholela. Through these efforts, staff put the earliest iterations of a health center practice that blended the social and medical sciences into action. Exploring outbreak control efforts therefore offers important insights into how the PCHC combined its research efforts and its program implementation and how it moved from the production of knowledge about a place to the actions necessary to improve health, and then how it measured success.

The annex from the 1951 Annual Report offers a useful and illustrative explanation of this process in its description of a two-month effort to control a typhoid outbreak in the region. Though later in the health center's tenure, it is representative of earlier efforts. In 1951, the health center received word that a number of people in a community called Hlabeni had fallen ill with typhoid. This particular community was outside of the PCHC's Designated Area, which meant that the doctor, medical aide, and health assistant, who made up the team that responded, had to start their outbreak control effort from scratch.

The team began at the hospital where the first known victim had been diagnosed with typhoid. They met with staff members who had attended the sick person and asked about the patient's illness and movements. The team learned that the first victim was a girl who attended a school ten miles from the farm where her family lived and worked. She had arrived at the hospital extremely sick with obvious signs of typhoid and had died less than a day after being admitted. The team knew that typhoid is a vector-borne illness that spreads through water sources or food contaminated by the excrement of a person carrying the *Salmonella enterica* serotype Typhi bacteria. This meant that the girl had to have contracted the illness by consuming contaminated food or water. The team therefore quickly began to retrace the movements of the patient, locating where she gathered water, where and what she ate, and where she went to the bathroom. The team hoped that her movements would lead them to the source of infection, which would help them stem the outbreak.

The team's efforts to piece together the girl's whereabouts in the days before her death led them to her school and home. In those places, they conducted interviews and learned that because of the distance between home and school, the girl stayed in the teachers' cottages during the week and went home only on weekends. The teachers told the team that upon arriving at school one Sunday, the girl had complained of a terrible headache and weakness; the next day, she returned home so her parents could care for her. Her parents explained that as the week progressed, her condition deteriorated. Finally, they took her to the hospital, where she died on Saturday, less than a week after her first symptoms appeared.

In this first case of the typhoid outbreak, the initial timeline (one week) and spatial extent of the disease (from farm to school to farm to hospital) was clear. In a matter of hours, the team had traced the girl's path and by extension the path of the bacteria across time and space through the people she interacted with. This was social medicine in action.[50] Through this methodical retracing, the team discovered a handful of other cases of typhoid from Hlabeni (the community with the school) and from another community called Ngwagane. In addition, following the social relationships and talking to teachers, family members, and nurses revealed that this was a very quick outbreak. Interviewees described rapid progression in the sick girl's body, in the population, and in the spaces she inhabited.

After the team had gathered data, they needed to organize, display, and analyze the information in order to make the outbreak legible to the outside world and to make a plan to combat it. They did so in two ways: First, using a community map created with the aid of a compass and their ever-increasing knowledge of the area, the health assistants detailed homesteads and water sources (potential sites of infection) as they were arrayed in the community in cartographic space on a piece of paper. As one of the maps from the 1951 outbreak reveals, they then added pertinent information, in this case an "X" to mark homesteads where typhoid cases had been confirmed, and a red arrow to note the direction of movement and spread (see figures 1.3 and 1.4). Just as with the maps of the community in the Designated Area, this map showed a community made up of households, water sources, and other buildings. But this map differed because it included water sources, infected households, and movement. As a result, it told the story of the outbreak. Indeed, by locating infection points spatially and by noting homesteads' relationships to each other and to their water sources, the health center offered a clear picture of the epidemic, where it began, where it might be going next, and how best to contain it. This way of understanding the spread of disease imposed a spatial vision over

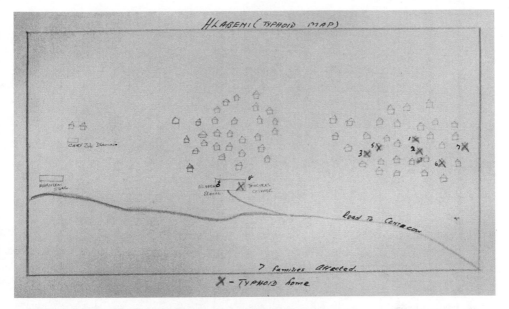

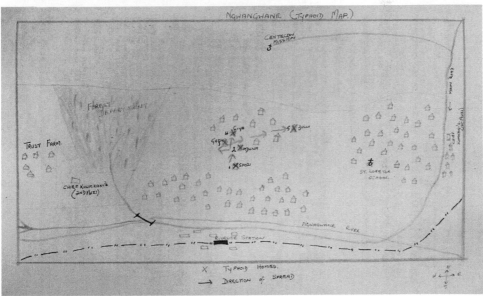

Figures 1.3 and 1.4 Typhoid map from the outbreak. 1951 Annual Report, SAB, GES vol. 1917, ref. 46/32.

the community where homesteads, orientation to water sources, and the movement of ill people became the most important features of the landscape. It also highlighted the inextricability of social relationships and biological agents for the spread of typhoid, mapping the movement of the two together. As such, these maps represented the combination of the spatial articulation of family and livelihood connections (social life) and medical understandings of the spatial pathology of typhoid bacteria (biological life). They also offered a roadmap, quite literally, for intervention. These maps were therefore the sites where social medicine's understanding of the important features of social life for health became legible as they were translated into practice.[51]

In addition to the maps, the health center described its outbreak control efforts through a narrative, borrowing from the technique it had developed from the family file and the case study. In this narrative, the author of the report arranged the paragraphs in a spatiotemporal order, taking the reader from family to family over time and across space as typhoid spread. Each paragraph focuses on a single family, the path of illness within the family, the symptoms various individuals reported, the treatment sought and received, and the outcome of the treatment. While some paragraphs include information about the distance between homesteads of an extended family or the migration patterns of individuals, the homestead and the family that occupy the paragraph remain intact and provide the anchor for the report's narrative structure. This particular presentation of the information the health center collected combines clinical observation, biomedical understandings of typhoid, the spatial layout of communities, familial relationships, and the stories health center staff collected from Hlabeni's residents, rooting them all in the household. The analysis offers the reader a picture of typhoid as a disease that moves from household to household, working its way through families and the individuals that make them up. This narrative pairs with the health center's outbreak maps, in which individual homesteads are a key part of the landscape and red arrows are used to show the movement of disease from one homestead to the next. This household-centered rendering of the typhoid outbreak led to a control effort that also centered on the household to improve health at the community scale. Like the community survey and family file, this story of the outbreak made it seem almost inevitable that control efforts would focus on the household, as again the household is the primary scale for social medicine.

The health center's research in Hlabeni and the maps it produced combined with knowledge about typhoid and how it spread to shape control efforts.[52] Health center staff treated sick individuals and inoculated family and community members who were not sick, but who had likely come into contact with the disease. The team visited households to encourage people to avoid particular watercourses, to protect clean ones, and to maintain good hygiene and defecate at a distance from food and water. They also taught them about typhoid, how it spreads, how it is treated, and how best to prevent it. Thanks to the qualitative social science research health center personnel conducted, these interventions were targeted, focusing on those households most affected or most likely to be affected by the disease in order to stem the outbreak in the community. The practice of outbreak control represented the coming together of qualitative social science, quantitative social science, and biomedicine; it was the earliest incarnation of the PCHC's program of social medicine.[53]

Seeing Like a Health Center

To see like a health center was to see the social life of Pholela through the quantitative and qualitative social sciences. It was to make Pholela, its people, and their health legible through surveys, analysis, interviews, and stories. To see like a health center was to impose an order on life in Pholela while at the same time recognizing how complex social medicine would need to be in practice. This vision grew out of the lecture halls of the University of the Witwatersrand's most progressive professors, was based in Kark and Jali's experience with the Bantu Nutrition Survey, and was rooted in what would be called today anti-racist progressive politics. It reflected a broad-based concern about equal access to health care, poverty, and inequality, the conviction that health and poverty are deeply intertwined, and a commitment to blending qualitative and quantitative social science methods with biomedical methods. Further, contending that ill health in Pholela and South Africa as a whole was about community-wide health more than individual health, the PCHC developed a social medicine practice focused on and located in Pholela's communities and households, rather than in the clinic. Scientific practices including biomedicine, epidemiology, cartography, and social sciences like anthropology made the endeavor possible by helping to define the communities and households in which the practices would be enacted. This was the first step toward implementing social medicine. It was also a world-making process where the world of health and healing that the health center would intervene in could be understood through science.

This newly forming scientific practice of social medicine also needed a way to connect people, diseases, homes, and political economy to each other predictably. The scalar hierarchy of individual, household, community, and nation that the PCHC developed did just that. Through their medical school training in biomedicine, the Karks understood how health and illness manifest in the biology of individual bodies. Through their training in the social sciences, they had learned about the political-economic structures that shape life, livelihoods, and health on a national scale. The household and the community scales became crucial for connecting the individual of biomedicine to the nation of social science. The hierarchical scalar structure the PCHC mapped onto Pholela enabled a practice of social medicine that was multiscalar at its heart, treating individuals as members of families in the clinic and intervening in the homesteads of the Designated Area to improve the health of the community, all while attending to the political-economic structures of the nation. To see like a health center was to see these four well-defined scales and to recognize their entanglements.

While this vision enabled the development of a practice that would be legible and replicable beyond Pholela, the reality of health and illness was much more complicated. The health center's efforts to stem the Hlabeni typhoid outbreak is an example of this. In the narrative of the outbreak, the story of the household-by-household progression quickly breaks down. When one reads the paragraphs or the more note-like explanations that accompany them, one sees that the people who made up these households and families visited different communities, attended schools away from their homes, and sought treatment in unexpected places at a distance. The spatially circumscribed outbreak maps and the neat progression of the history of the epidemic as moving from the space of one household to the space of the next distorts the complicated travel patterns of area residents, a livelihood strategy that moved beyond community boundaries, and the pathogens residents carried in their bodies. This messy reality challenged the scalar hierarchy of health center practice.

There are hints of this in the report itself: there is a discussion of the mass inoculation of a missionary community because a boy sick with typhoid had rented a room there, and there is a rather perplexed paragraph on water supply where the health center staff explain that they could not find a common source for typhoid in Hlabeni. But overall, the story of the typhoid outbreak is the story of multiscalar social science in action. As such, it is an example of what it takes to make a place and practice legible to the outside world. Taken as a whole, the report reveals the work the health center team did to organize the outbreak to fit a particular framework, as well as the necessity of grappling with a reality that does not fit that framework. The bulleted sidebar notes reveal that outbreaks can be messy and that scale is always constructed.[54] This complexity challenges the neat legible practice the health center created through its surveying and mapping efforts. It also had implications for social medicine, at least in practice.

The outbreak control team's success rested on their willingness to follow people and their relationships, whether or not they fit into the scalar model the health center staff arrived with and wrote about. The health center's willingness to modify its social medicine practice to fit the circumstances of the outbreak worked. In Hlabeni, in less than two months, the team had fully contained the outbreak. The results were impressive: only three people died and just fifteen were hospitalized. Many people had been successfully treated at home, and the vast majority had been immunized to prevent infection in the future. In short, thanks to the PCHC team's quick investigation, one that followed a biological agent through social relationships, and thanks to its control efforts, this potentially serious outbreak had been successfully contained.[55] Its approach was so successful that by the middle of the 1940s, government officials asked the health center's team to help stem outbreaks throughout the area and as far away as Pietermaritzburg, a major city and the provincial capital, with a far more advanced public health infrastructure.[56] Even more telling, this particular technique, pioneered in Pholela, was eventually replicated throughout all of South Africa.[57]

Enacting social medicine and seeing like a health center meant two interconnected things: making the health center practice legible and reorganizing social life in Pholela to fit its spatial logic. First, it meant making people, places, livelihoods, health, and health center practice legible so that the PCHC and its supporters could see its successes. This lesson is, in some ways, a logical extension of the scholarship about producing scientific knowledge and producing modern states. In order to know a place, its people, their health, and their environment *scientifically*, complexity must be simplified; this is an important precursor to making that place legible. Making the PCHC's work legible required a number of steps: teaching and enacting social medicine, mapping people, places, and diseases, and enumerating households and populations. This enabled the health center to render community health visible through epidemiological analysis. Second, enacting social medicine meant reorganizing social life in Pholela to fit a particular spatial logic, while in practice grappling with the complex social reality of life, livelihoods, and health in order to improve them all. But enacting social medicine also meant telling complex stories based on information collected in the family file and enacting a practice that attended as much to the messy reality of life as it did to the spatial organization the health center had mapped onto communities. The cases of the woman with syphilis and the Hlabeni typhoid outbreak were evidence of this. In both instances, to see like a health center was to define units for analysis and intervention, making them a reality through practice, but it was also to transgress that model when necessary to treat individuals or communities, and to improve health. Through its practice, the PCHC recognized that reality was complex, and practice and vision did not always align. Seeing like a health center meant making certain aspects of health center practice visible to the outside world, all while recognizing how very constructed those aspects and the scientific knowledge that underlay them were in practice.

2

Relationships and Social Medicine

On a crisp fall day in 2008, I was sitting on a bench in the yard belonging to one of the *gogos* I would come to visit regularly. Warmed by the late afternoon sun, we were having a relaxed conversation about what life was like in her community, Enkangala, in her youth. I was new to research and self-conscious about everything I didn't know. Talking with Gogo Sithole, then eighty-three years old, about her childhood memories offered one way to understand the second quarter of the twentieth century, the period just before and at the start of the PCHC. This first interview was important, not just for the information I learned, but also because it began to lay the groundwork for what was to become one of the most important relationships for my research and my life in Pholela.

As our interview progressed, I quickly learned that Gogo was an old hand at research. Her experience with the PCHC in the 1940s and 1950s had taught her much about the process of social science research, her role as a research participant, and the job of the researcher. In this first long interview with Gogo Sithole and in many subsequent interviews, I learned an important lesson: the data, analysis, and publications that the PCHC and its staff produced from the work they did in Pholela—the social medicine they developed—required a good deal of effort on the part of area residents and rested on their relationships with health center staff.

Several months after my first interview with Gogo Sithole, I was back at her home. I had been in the South African National Archives and the Historical Papers Research Archive at the University of the Witwatersrand for several weeks. When I returned to Pholela, the health extension work of the PCHC was at the forefront of my mind. Though I had been to Gogo Sithole's home many times, it felt like I was observing with fresh eyes. I began to notice various elements like the vegetable garden, pit latrines, and rubbish pit that I had been learning about in the archives. These elements had been central to the health center's vision of a healthy homestead and by extension social medicine. As we ambled about chatting, I looked down and right in front of us was a new water tap; I asked Gogo about it. She told me that the family had pooled its money to buy a new tap because their other one had run dry. Access to protected water was important, as Gogo Sithole and her neighbors had explained to me, because it ensured that they would not get sick from bacteria in the water they drank. As I had been learning, in the years before the PCHC, there were no protected water sources in Pholela, nor were there pit latrines, rubbish pits, compost pits, or diverse gardens. Walking around Gogo Sithole's homestead that afternoon, it suddenly dawned on me that many of the homestead elements I had taken for granted were actually products of the health center's social medicine program and that they remained thanks to the upkeep of Pholela's residents.

In order for the health center to succeed, it needed Pholela's residents to participate. Residents had to learn how to be good research subjects by understanding what researchers were looking for and by learning how to answer questions. They also needed to take the health center's advice and modify their homesteads. In return, they would come to play an important role in shaping the data collected, the analysis produced, and the practices that followed. Through this, they were integral to COPC as it developed in Pholela. This point may seem obvious: of course the people who participate in research play a role in outcomes. But research subjects also play an important role in the production of *researchers* and, in Pholela, they played a role in the production of social medicine practitioners too.[1] COPC and its success also depended on the things of health center work: seeds, pits, taps, and windows. Together, residents and health center staff enacted social medicine through these things as assemblages of humans and nonhumans became as important to the social medicine developed in Pholela and its success as relationships among people were.

This chapter, anchored in Pholela's homesteads, in my experience as a researcher, and in Gogo Sithole's and her neighbors' experiences as research subjects, reveals that seeing like a health center meant seeing, at least in part, through the eyes, homes, and lives of area residents, even if the health center did not recognize them as part of its vision. In enacting its social medicine program in Pholela, the PCHC reconfigured relationships, severing some (among bacteria, watercourses, and people, for example) and creating others (among health assistants, residents, nutrients, and healthy cells, for example). Together, these things and people transformed homestead landscapes and health in Pholela. And yet these relationships remained largely invisible, even though they became the foundation of social medicine, acting as both cause and effect in the creation of this new science. As Donald Moore argues, places are not simply stages upon which interactions unfold; they are topography and vegetation, buildings and gardens, all co-constituted through and with the actions of the people who inhabit them.[2] With this understanding of place in mind, social medicine from the homesteads of Pholela offers a different vision of social life, one where the relationships among residents, between residents and health center staff, and among people and things are fundamental; through a focus on the place of the homestead, nonhumans are as important to social life as humans. This was the social life that underpinned what would become the social medicine practice of COPC.

Learning to Do Research

As Gogo Sithole and I sat in her yard chatting the afternoon of our first major interview, her grandchildren and great grandchildren milled about the homestead, talking and joking, listening to popular Zulu gospel music, and playing with whatever stray ball, plastic tub, or stick lay about. Amid the activity, people yelled back and forth and neighbors and friends walked by greeting each other and Gogo Sithole. We talked casually about the PCHC in the "time of the Karks," a label she and her contemporaries gave to the period of 1940 to 1962 when the health center was fully operational. All of 5'1", Gogo Sithole sat next to me on the bench hunched over laughing as we talked, often poking fun at me, her family, and herself in response. In rather general terms, she explained how nice the Karks were and how important they had been to her and the rest of Pholela. Proudly, she told me that she had named her first daughter, Carol, after theirs.

After a few minutes, I pulled out the piece of paper on which I had printed the household history questions I would be asking all of the families in my study. I had based my questions on the publications of the PCHC, hoping to gather similar data so that I could trace change over time. Early in our conversation, it was clear that Gogo Sithole had an excellent memory. And, thanks to the fact that she had been employed as a domestic worker by the Karks, she had knowledge about the doctors and the work they did in Pholela that many of her generation did not. Moreover, she liked to talk and she was entirely unselfconscious.[3] While I was new to research, it seemed like these were good qualities to have in an interviewee.

Reading questions from the paper, I began pressing Gogo Sithole for more specific information. I had been taking notes since we sat down, but these new,

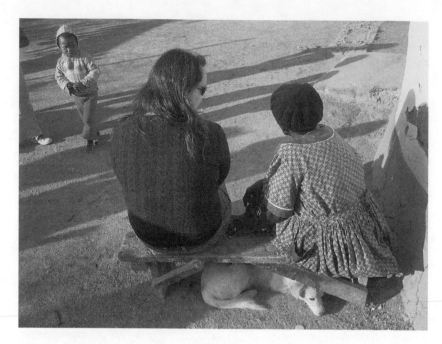

Figure 2.1 The author with Gogo Sithole. Photo by Saskia Wusterfeldt.

formal questions, and the paper from which I read them, signaled a shift. Gogo Sithole immediately picked up on this; she sat straighter and the wrinkles in the space between her eyebrows deepened as she concentrated in order to be sure that she fully understood what I was asking. The activity around us faded into the background, and when Gogo spoke, it was directly to me. Her answers were both accurate and comprehensible, two good qualities for research, it seemed to me. We had shifted to a formal interview. I fumbled a bit, trying to stay on top of the questions I thought I needed to ask, following up on what Gogo was saying, and furiously scribbling everything down.

We carried on like this for a few questions until Gogo Sithole stopped me. She told me she knew exactly what we were doing. She explained that in the "time of the Karks," health assistants and researchers would come around and ask many of the same kinds of questions. And then she pointed out that I wasn't doing it very well because I didn't know the right order of the questions and I didn't phrase them correctly. In addition, I fumbled a bit and I appeared unprepared (which was true, it being my first interview). To be the kind of researcher Gogo Sithole was expecting, I needed to ask the right kinds of questions—about specific illnesses, crop yields, and hygiene practices in the household—and I needed to do so quickly, efficiently, and confidently using the correct phrasing, all in the right order. In return, Gogo would answer those questions "correctly," concisely, and efficiently. Efficiency was a priority for good research, it seemed. In her experience, those were our roles in the research process. In this first encounter (and in many thereafter), Gogo Sithole was more than willing to let me know that I had not yet mastered what it meant to be a researcher.

This story of my first interview with Gogo Sithole stands out in my mind. Schooled in feminist research methods, I understood that interviews are conversations, and that relationships form the bedrock of social science research. And I was well aware that I had a lot of learning to do.[4] Still, I had not expected such direction from my interviewee. After all, many of the feminist scholars whom I was reading argued that the relationships between researchers and research subjects are situated in a hierarchical binary, where the researcher is in a position of power over the research subject, especially vis-à-vis the global terrain of power.[5] From the outside, our positions seemed to confirm this. I was and am a highly educated white woman from a university in the Global North, and Gogo was an uneducated African woman living in a mudbrick home without running water. To anyone observing, it would seem clear that I had more power than Gogo Sithole. In a strictly political-economic sense, this is true. And so, careful to reflect on my position, I thought I would be the one guiding our conversations and that I would need to consciously open up space for Gogo to share.[6] But this was not the case in Pholela. Gogo Sithole and the other gogos and *mkhulus* (grandpas) I worked with were often quite directive, instructing me on how to do research while simultaneously answering my questions. These residents set the tone of the research process and taught me what it meant to do research. Their guidance often made for a more efficient and consistent research practice on my part, both hallmarks of what I imagined to be "good" social science. Through these experiences, the impact of the PCHC's research practices fifty years prior was having a direct impact on mine.[7]

Developing a Practice of Social Medicine

For the PCHC, the surveys I described in the last chapter were particularly important to the relationships that underpinned social medicine, because they offered multiple opportunities for residents and health center staff to get to know each other and to learn how to do research together. In the beginning, people thought that the questions that the health assistants asked seemed strange and invasive. Residents explained that, as time went on, they started to understand what information the health assistants were looking for and therefore could answer more easily. As they became accustomed to the research process, the questions began to seem less invasive. This was often an anecdote offered to make me feel better about my own process in the beginning as I was stumbling over my questions and learning how to conduct research. But it also shows that to be successful, health center staff had to listen to residents, quickly learn about life in Pholela, and recognize their role in its social life. And the staff at the PCHC did, with remarkable skill.

For their part, residents quickly learned to give the right kind of information for the studies undertaken: how much milk (in pints) their cows produced or how many months a year the men were away. In other words, in order to be good research subjects, Pholela's residents came to understand that they were being asked if their house was a healthy place in scientific (social and biomedical) terms. Therefore, they needed to know not only what information was important, but also the form in which the health center wanted the information. Their answers, given in standard units, could then be compared and compounded, made into percentages in order to render communities comparable and to measure overall success (and failure). Standard units were key components of this research. But rather than something imposed by the health center, these units were negotiated by health center staff and Pholela's residents through research encounters. Long before the Karks came to Pholela, residents knew how much they grew or how much milk their cow(s) produced. As a result, the early research process was more about finding a standard measurement that worked for residents than it was about making Pholela and its people fit into a predetermined standard that would be legible beyond Pholela.[8]

Once the first survey was complete, the health center began its health extension work, pairing its surveys and research projects with education in an effort to improve health. Knowledge gained through health education made residents better able to answer questions, thereby improving the speed and accuracy of research, as health education fed back into research. At the same time, this knowledge ensured that residents understood what information the health assistants were looking for and could thereby answer questions "correctly," regardless of whether or not their answers matched reality. For example, many of the gogos in Pholela recall that women, and especially members of the maternal and child welfare program, visited the clinic regularly to have their babies examined. When they went to the clinic, the doctors asked them if they had been to the *inyanga*.[9] The women would say no, since they knew that was what the health center wanted to hear, even though they were, for the most part, all visiting an inyanga for important preventive health treatments for their babies.[10] These women knew the "correct" answer and so they gave it, regardless of whether it matched their actual behavior. In return, the health

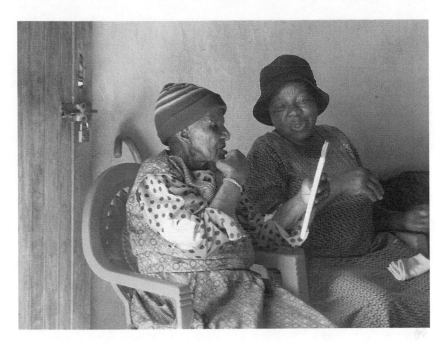

Figure 2.2 Gogo Sithole takes over the role of the researcher. Photo by author.

center was able to report their impressive successes in getting residents to abandon what they saw as harmful healing practices in favor of scientific medicine. This "success" then helped to ensure ongoing funding.

The role of residents in shaping research through their answers was also visible in archival documents. For example, early reports revealed that at first some residents resisted government agents (in this case, health center staff) going door-to-door to collect information. As one early newspaper article put it, "The start was not auspicious. The Natives were un-co-operative and an attempt to supply the whole area with health services showed no measurable results."[11] Indeed, many documents from the 1940s and 1950s lament that some residents continued to refuse to participate. Tinged with judgment, they mention how those who did not participate were lazy, uneducated people who held onto their "superstitious beliefs," to their detriment. According to the PCHC, this persistent "ignorance" had a heavy price, resulting in illness and death.[12] While this rendering reveals much about what the health center thought about those who did not participate, at least in its official publications, it also reveals that in spite of its rousing success, the PCHC never managed to enroll everyone in its Designated Area. Scholars like James Scott, Susan Leigh Star, and Martha Lampland remind us that standardization is never totalizing and can never capture the full texture of life. As the example the gogos gave reveals, research subjects don't always give accurate answers. Sometimes this is an act of resistance and sometimes it is because their lives do not fit standardized models.[13] The bottom line is that data and statistics are not a clear and complete rendering of the world as it is. Neither were the family files, nor the case studies, for that matter. It is important not to overstate this. From residents' accounts and PCHC accounts, the vast majority of questions were straightforward and resulted in accurate answers. Nonetheless, the conclusions that the PCHC reached from their data were always partial.

As the PCHC began to develop COPC in the 1940s, residents faced a new way of seeing, understanding, and measuring the world, just as health center staff faced a landscape and people who were new and unfamiliar. Together, they developed a research and social medicine practice and the tools with which to implement it. This practice did not always measure life with complete accuracy, but it did represent knowledge that residents and staff produced together. Just as in the case of the HIV/AIDS research that Biruk describes, the standards used, data gathered, and social medicine practices developed in Pholela were the product of negotiations that came from the relationships between the PCHC and Pholela's residents.[14] Because the health center was interested in tracking epidemiological shifts over an extended period, health assistants resurveyed areas every year. As a result, the impact of these negotiations compounded. Through this process, the research subjects and the answers they provided had a tremendous impact on both the quality of the research produced and the results the PCHC wrote about. Whether or not it was conscious, the health center staff recognized this and understood that the best way to ensure quality was to develop positive and productive relationships with Pholela's residents. As a result, COPC and the publications health center doctors wrote about it were the product of the relationships between the people who lived in Pholela and the researchers who developed COPC.[15]

Relationships and Research Methods

When I developed the methodology for the research that I write about here, I had been learning about the PCHC's approach to data collection and analysis through the many publications from Pholela and about COPC. Rooted in the quantitative social sciences, the health center's method was concerned with legibility, standardization, replicability, and consistency. It also centered on the homestead as the locus for the family. Therefore, so was I. Even for my most in-depth research—the household histories—I chose eight families from three different communities to reduce "bias" in my results. And I chose the household because I was interested in people, practices, livelihoods, and the home landscape. The household seemed to be the best unit for the interviews and oral histories that would enable me to get at that information. As I conducted my research, I used the exact same set of questions with each household and for each date I was researching. This, I believed, would go a long way toward the standardization and replicability that I saw as the hallmark of the PCHC's research efforts and that seemed so important to "rigorous" social science research. It didn't take me long to realize that not only was replicability likely impossible; it was also undesirable. Instead, it was the complexity, richness, and difference of various encounters that emerged thanks to the relationships I was building with my research subjects that were important for understanding social medicine from Pholela.

Richness and complexity are hard to grasp. They take time, a depth of knowledge, and an intimacy with a place and its people. The visits and time Thokozile and I spent with our research subjects allowed us to develop the close, personal relationships that would help us understand the complexity of the place. Likewise, the PCHC's regular home visits for research and for education gave both health assistants and residents plenty of opportunities to get to know each other, to learn about surveys, and to learn their respective roles in the research process. As the Karks wrote, "The health team was getting to know the people in a more comprehensive way and becoming more conscious of their social, cultural, and belief systems in relation to their health. The community itself was becoming increasingly involved and participant in many health-related activities."[16] Feminist scholars have noted that relationships are the bedrock of much social science research. Tracing the development of COPC from its earliest days in Pholela reveals that relationships don't just underpin research, they also produce researchers. The Karks were not social medicine researchers before they began working with Pholela's residents, and Pholela's residents were not research subjects before the PCHC was established; they came into being together, through their multiple encounters. Long-term, engaged research changes everyone involved.[17] Likewise, research emerged through these encounters. As J.-K. Gibson-Graham write, and as I experienced, through the relationships built from research encounters, a common ground is possible and a research project emerges.[18] The same was certainly true in Pholela, where COPC emerged from the work the PCHC staff and area residents did together.

Reflexivity refers to the practice of the researcher reflecting on their positionality and how it affects research; long before it entered the research lexicon, the PCHC's staff was actively thinking about what they could do to mitigate power differences in Pholela by reflecting on their positionality and how it affected their work. They did so in an effort to better understand the community and to establish a medical practice best suited to it.[19] Residents remark that they saw that the health assistants, and the health center more generally, were adapting to Pholela. They often commented about how well they knew the health assistants because of frequent home visits. They spoke of how helpful and nice the health assistants were, and, most importantly, they mentioned that the health center listened to and learned from them. Residents remark that the health center staff cared about what the community had to say. The PCHC's social medicine practice, rooted in long-term research and relationships, was embedded in the complexity of life in Pholela, even as its survey work sought to simplify that life. The family files and the case write-ups that came from them are evidence of the textured understanding the PCHC achieved—an understanding that can only come from mutual respect and trust. This approach is a hallmark of feminist research. As Audrey Kobayashi writes, feminist researchers "require research methods that recognize the relationship with others as one of (ideally) mutual concern and trust."[20] This book, both in terms of the PCHC data it draws on and in terms of my own ethnographic method, is testament to these relationships.

Over the years, as I listened to Gogo Sithole, one thing that always stood out was her profound affection for the PCHC staff and the Karks in particular. She was not alone. In conversation after conversation, it was clear that the people of Pholela cherished their relationships with the Karks, John Cassel, and the doctors who followed them. This was, of course, in part because of the prestige the PCHC had brought to this place, the resources it had, and the health improvements it catalyzed, not to mention the cultural currency that proximity to whiteness brings in a place so heavily marked by racial capitalism. But it was also because the PCHC staff members were their friends. The social medicine practiced in Pholela had fostered new relationships, and those relationships remained important even decades later. When I first started my research, one woman, a retired nurse, asked me if I knew Emily Kark. She had received a Christmas card for years but hadn't gotten one in the previous couple of years and was worried about her friend. These relationships of mutual concern and care were crucial for the work and success of the health center. As Kim England notes in her writing about qualitative research, the health center and Pholela's residents had reciprocal relationships, built on mutual concern and trust.[21] Through these relationships, they built a new brand of social medicine, one in which the contributions of Pholela's African residents, the majority of whom lived in poverty, were as important as those of the highly trained doctors.

Enacting Social Medicine: Remaking the Homestead

Relationships among people were not the only ones that mattered in Pholela; things mattered too. Once the first phases of research and education were complete, the health center began its efforts to improve health and prevent illness in communities with a focus on the homestead. To make the homestead a healthy place, the PCHC believed that residents needed to add new elements, rearrange existing components, and keep everything neat and tidy; they needed to reshape the landscape. Successfully remaking the homestead required that health assistants and residents work together and learn from each other, as the family took charge of protecting its own health. It also required new assemblages of people and things, as together, health assistants and Pholela's residents reconfigured relationships through health center work. The concept of the assemblage provides a useful way to think about the relationships among humans and nonhumans because it recognizes that humans and nonhumans act together without prescribing how their relationships work. As such, assemblages allow for an understanding that bacteria, water, people, and political economy act together to make someone sick with a waterborne illness without determining exactly how they come together. In addition, assemblages can interact to form and reform each other. In so doing, human–nonhuman assemblages help reform other social relationships like those between Pholela's residents and the state.[22] Through new assemblages of human and nonhuman relationships, the place of the homestead and its landscape changed, and so did health.

Central to the PCHC's plan to remake the homestead was the creation of a new waste disposal system: a compost pit to fertilize the home garden, a rubbish pit to burn regularly, and a pit latrine for the disposal of human waste.[23] This three-part system sought to standardize waste removal and keep pathogens away from people in order to prevent diseases from spreading. Drawing on what it had learned through its early efforts to stem outbreaks of diseases like typhoid, the health center reasoned that when built, the rubbish pit would lead to fewer flies, which bred in the garbage that lay in the yard; and a pit latrine would keep the flies that remained away from human waste, thereby preventing them from transporting *Salmonella typhi* to the food residents ate. For added protection, health assistants encouraged residents to cover food to keep any remaining flies and the diseases they might carry from touching it, just in case the waste disposal system was not 100 percent effective. Taken together, these simple alterations to the homestead would prevent the outbreaks the health center had worked so hard to stem.

To prevent other illnesses like flu or tuberculosis, health assistants enacted other plans to keep germs away from people. They encouraged residents to modify buildings to improve ventilation, replacing permanent windows with ones that opened, enlarging others, and adding more.[24] The health center believed that these changes would reduce the number of bacteria or virus particles in the air, thereby making it harder for TB and flu to spread. The health center also pushed residents to clean buildings and homesteads regularly to ensure that vermin like the insects and rodents that carried scabies or certain fevers did not populate the same spaces as people. Similarly, centralizing rubbish disposal and burning it regularly meant that there was no longer any place for vermin like rats to hide. These steps, the PCHC believed, were key to a healthy family. In short, in applying the best public health and biomedical practices of the time, the PCHC sought to separate people from germs. As one resident recalled, "Dr. Kark came to teach people that every disease had a cause and that that cause was a sort of bacteria."[25] By this logic, in order for the PCHC to succeed, people had to be kept apart from "bacteria" (here a term referring to any and all pathogens), and the bacteria that led to a disease needed to be kept from spreading in the landscape; a well-ordered and clean homestead would do just that.

Of course, the PCHC understood ill health to be rooted in social structures as well. For the health center, South Africa's system of racial capitalism, which kept Africans in the Reserves and ensured that they would remain destitute, was the ultimate social cause of illness. But these broad-scale political-economic processes were harder, if not impossible, to intervene in. As a result, the PCHC saw efforts to remake homesteads as purely biomedical. They were a winnable stopgap measure (an intervention in the biological world) that could improve health, even if they did not reduce poverty (the most important aspect of the social world). By locating disease in the physical and biological environment, and by separating disease from people, the health center situated these nonhumans outside of the social world of Pholela's residents. This approach of focusing narrowly on the biological was quite successful. As chapter 1 details, typhoid and other infectious disease epidemics all but disappeared and overall health improved markedly. The separation of people from germs was making for healthier people, at least in biomedical terms.

Disease prevention was only one aspect of the health center's program in homesteads. Health promotion was also important. To promote health, the PCHC focused on the home vegetable garden, which is the focus of the next chapter. Thanks in part to Sydney Kark's and Edward Jali's work on the Bantu nutrition survey, the health center saw vegetables packed with vitamins and minerals (micronutrients) as key to improving baseline health. The homestead vegetable garden became an important component of COPC because it was seen as an easy way to supply nutrients to residents' diets. Building gardens and growing new crops required new seeds, new tools and techniques, new knowledge, and labor, especially at first. As a result, health assistants and Pholela's residents built these home vegetable gardens together, with seeds and tools provided by the health center and tips and techniques offered by agricultural extension workers in the area. Once vegetables began growing, residents consumed them from their gardens. The micronutrients in those vegetables helped to counteract some of the most pernicious aspects of malnutrition and led to significant drops in overall rates. In this example, with the help of health assistants, residents incorporated the vegetables they grew into their diets and their bodies, and the nutrients in those vegetables helped to improve cellular development and overall health in ways anticipated by nutritional science. Again, this was a biomedical solution to a health problem. It was an intervention in the biology of the landscape, but just as in the case of the new waste-disposal system, it was an intervention that necessarily involved people. Vegetables, people, nutrients, cells, and science all worked together to improve health. These improvements in health motivated residents to continue planting vegetables as they felt their positive effects and saw them in their children. Thanks to the impact that increased nutrients in diets had on residents, the nonhuman components of gardens like soil, seeds, and shovels became integral to the relationships between health center staff and residents that underpinned the COPC developing in Pholela. Through assemblages of human and nonhuman actors that produced new vegetable gardens, the homestead landscape and the bodies of Pholela's resident were transformed.

The new assemblages built through homestead transformation catalyzed even more new relationships. Soon after they began planting new vegetables in their home gardens, Pholela's women formed seed cooperatives to share seeds and knowledge as they worked to improve their gardens in terms of both taste and nutrition. As women traded seeds, their gardens grew more diverse and their yields improved. Together, the women in the cooperatives selected vegetables and seeds for taste and productivity. These seeds, the vegetables they would become, and the nutrients they would supply led to a new social formation and more influence for the women of Pholela beyond their gardens. The seed cooperatives became the basis for a women's advisory group, first at the health center and later for the chief, as women gained an official voice in formal politics. The new social organization around seeds mattered beyond Pholela too. As the women who were members of the seed cooperatives interacted with health center staff, the PCHC began to see the positive impact that these cooperatives offered garden variety and yields. Seeing this as an excellent community solution to a health problem (malnutrition), the Karks and others incorporated cooperatives into COPC. By the 1970s, seed and other cooperatives had become a hallmark of this brand of social medicine as they traveled beyond Pholela to places like Mound Bayou, Mississippi. In Mound Bayou, the site of the first rural health center modeled on Pholela in the United States, the farmers' cooperative was one of its most important and distinctive features.[26]

The PCHC staff's ability to recognize the value of seed cooperatives and their subsequent incorporation into COPC was thanks to the staff's relationships with Pholela's women. But that was not all; the value of these cooperatives came in part through the seeds the women shared, the vegetables that grew from them, and the nutrients they contained. After all, it was improvements in health that the health center cared most about. In their examination of the Zimbabwean bush pump and the social relations it shapes, Marianne de Laet and Annemarie Mol explain that the success of the bush pump was a result of its fluidity—its ability to adapt to the particular context and relationships it was embedded in—and, moreover, its ability to take on the characteristics of its different environments.[27] The seed cooperatives that became integral to COPC represented the same kind of fluid technology. They adapted to new contexts and enabled place-specific configurations of the human–nonhuman relationships necessary to their own success. For example, in Mound Bayou, there was a large-scale farming cooperative that grew vegetables appropriate for the climate of the delta and men were often in charge. As a result of the flexibility of the cooperative model, the seeds these women shared led to new configurations of human social relationships that would extend beyond Pholela to other sites of COPC and beyond gardens to broader political structures. It would not be a stretch to say that thanks to the flexibility of the seed cooperative model, residents like Gogo Sithole have left a mark on places like Mound Bayou, Mississippi, and Jerusalem. It was the nonhumans that made it possible for Pholela's women to leave this mark because these things could travel.

As the example of seed cooperatives and gardens reveals, the social relationships that included people and things underlie the dramatic improvements in the health and the groundbreaking innovations the PCHC offered social medicine. These relationships are obscured by the aggregate data that fill annual reports, articles, and books written about the PCHC, rendered invisible in official accounts of COPC. In their role as research subjects and in their relationships with researchers and the things of social medicine, Pholela's residents and their knowledge, experience, and social world had a tremendous impact on how the PCHC, the government, and the rest of the world would understand Pholela and replicate the social medicine developed there.

An examination of health center practice opens up the question of who and what counts as social. For the health center, the program of remaking the homestead was always about the biology of health. It was a project the health center could complete (with residents) to improve health because the social problems seemed insurmountable. As a result, many nonhumans, like vegetables, also set the terms for success. It is important to recognize the role of the new homestead landscape and the things that populated it in the success of social medicine; without them, little would have changed. But those things could never act alone. Residents needed to use them and build them, and the health center needed to provide and teach about them. Through its efforts to reorganize the homestead landscape, the PCHC helped to reorder the relationships among homestead elements and between people and things, creating new assemblages and disassembling others. Attending to the construction of landscapes reveals that seeds and nutrients, windows and bacteria, and their relationships with each other and with people, all shaped the successes and failures of social medicine in Pholela. This understanding of social life is a radical departure from a view focused solely on people. In this telling, as Jane Bennett explains, things play a role in shaping the world just as people do.[28] Once things are recognized as "vital" players, social life must expand beyond the human. As Bruno Latour explains in *Reassembling the Social*, the "social" is both nowhere in particular and everywhere, as it connects people and things which interact with each other as they *"make others do things."*[29] Nutrients make people plant new vegetable seeds and typhoid makes people centralize waste. In the homesteads of Pholela's residents, people (residents and health assistants) and things (pits and the shovels to dig them, vegetables, their nutrients, and lessons in agriculture and nutrition) worked together to transform homesteads into healthier places and, by extension, to turn people into healthier individuals. As Sara Ahmed writes, "[W]hile bodies do things, things might also 'do bodies.'"[30] The seeds shared through women-led cooperatives that became the vegetables that Pholela's residents ingested helped make healthier bodies. These seeds (the things) and the human relationships that got them into gardens and cooking pots made for healthier people. And those people, counted in households and summed at the community scale, became evidence of the efficacy of social medicine. It was the assemblages of people and things that provided for that evidence in the first place.

Relationships and Social Medicine

New assemblages and relationships among people and between people and things constituted the social fabric of health center work. Lyn Schumaker writes that the importance of relationships among researchers and research subjects lay "in their usefulness for anthropological activity."[31] In her research on the history of the Rhodes-Livingston Institute (RLI), the most prolific anthropological research center in Africa, she found that it was the relationships between researchers and research subjects that not only underpinned the research produced, but were the foundation for anthropology more broadly. Expanding this idea beyond the human, Bruce Braun writes that understanding the world as more than human stems from "the assumption that social life—indeed all life—is an outcome of complex assemblages in which humans are not the only actors."[32] As Braun points out, nonhumans are important social actors too. In Pholela, nonhumans made up homesteads along with humans and played an important role in the formation of social medicine; it was out of these human–nonhuman assemblages that social medicine grew. In this accounting of social medicine from Pholela, human–nonhuman relationships make up social life. Yet, for the PCHC, social life continued to be understood through the social sciences. As a result, the relationships upon which its success and its practice rested remained largely invisible. Nevertheless, as became clear to me sitting in Gogo Sithole's homestead and learning about research and about the PCHC, relationships among people and human–nonhuman assemblages constituted in the homestead underpinned the social medicine developed in Pholela. The neat division of the social sciences and the biomedical sciences through which the health center understood Pholela obscured this fact.

The value of writing from Pholela, from the perspective of this place and its people, is that it centers relationships. Social medicine from Pholela is rooted in the human–nonhuman assemblages that make up this place. My experience in Pholela and relationships with residents taught me this. As Marilyn Strathern writes, "it is through their relations with others that [researchers] understand relationships."[33] And as Gillian Rose writes, one of the consequences of these relationships is that "neither the researcher nor the researched remains unchanged through the research encounter."[34] As the story of my interview with Gogo Sithole makes clear, the woman I met and worked with was forever shaped by her relationships with the people who worked at the PCHC. The PCHC's practice produced research subjects. Its work in communities also produced researchers, as the health center's staff learned how to be social medicine practitioners through their work with Pholela's residents (just as I learned how to be a researcher through my work with Gogo Sithole and her neighbors). In her study of the RLI, Schumaker asserts that relationships between British researchers and African researchers ensured that anthropology would be "an activity done by and meaningful to Africans."[35] Likewise, thanks to the long-term relationships developed in Pholela, within a few years, the work at and by the PCHC was largely carried out by community members and, as my interviews with older residents attest, was deeply meaningful to the community, to the homestead landscape, and to the individuals whose health improved. But the PCHC's social medicine was not just meaningful to Pholela's residents; it was also the *product* of their relationships with the staff at the PCHC and the things of social medicine.

Science studies scholars have long sought to uncover the social relationships that underpin science. As Sandra Harding writes, science is "co-constituted with [its] social [order]."[36] Through insights like this one, feminist and postcolonial scholars have challenged often unspoken assumptions that science is a white, male endeavor. In doing so, they question ideas of universality and objectivity—ideas that are entangled with the practices of legibility, standardization, replicability, and consistency that were so important in the survey work in Pholela. These scholars demonstrate that objectivity and universality are partial and particular, and that science is as much about the places in which research is conducted and the people it is conducted by and with as it is about the subjects researched and knowledge produced.[37] In Pholela and in many places in the Global South, the relationships that formed the basis of the practice of science are obscured. The result is that people like Gogo Sithole are written out of the stories of scientific achievement. Twenty minutes sitting on a bench in Gogo Sithole's yard taught me how important that silence is. But sitting in her yard also taught me that things matter. Donna Haraway and others demonstrate that nonhumans play an important role in the practices of science, the production of knowledge, and everyday life more generally. Taken together, these scholars demonstrate that knowledge, practices, landscapes, and people are the products of assemblages of people, plants, animals, and things.[38]

3

Nutrition, Science, and Racial Capitalism

When the Karks arrived in Pholela, they saw malnutrition even before they examined their first patients.[1] As they visited homesteads, they met small women, men, girls, and boys; many had distended bellies, reddish hair, and lighter patches of skin on their arms, legs, and faces. These were all telltale signs of nutrient deficiencies.[2] The health center team quickly learned that where Pholela's residents got their food and by extension their nutrition was complicated. Residents employed a mixed livelihood strategy which they had developed in response to the lack of sufficient land and labor in Pholela. Because of the connection between livelihoods and food, the health center viewed malnutrition as not simply a health problem, but as evidence of a more complete failure of social life in South Africa.

The PCHC's staff understood that the social forces shaping malnutrition were the political-economic forces shaping the livelihoods of households and structuring the nation's economy. And because malnutrition was wrapped up in larger failures of political economy, so too was health.[3] While the health center staff recognized that they could do little about the way racial capitalism structured life and opportunity in South Africa, they believed that they could do something about household livelihoods, particularly related to food consumption. There began the nutrition program.

In South Africa as a whole, and in Pholela specifically, nutrition was the prism through which government officials and health center personnel understood health in a context of poverty. Through nutrition, social life and the biological body came together; this was perfect for social medicine.[4] As one of South Africa's highest officials for Native Affairs, the chief native commissioner, wrote, "Malnutrition is recognized as one of the chief causes of ill-health among Natives today, particularly children. . . . A Health Scheme would be of no value without taking into account measures for proper and adequate food supplies."[5] In Pholela, the nutrition program became the centerpiece of the health center's efforts. It had two parts. First, the health center used the "Grow and Eat More Vegetables" campaign to increase the micronutrients in residents' diets by getting them to "Grow and Eat" new, micronutrient-packed vegetables. Second, the health center set up a program to increase protein consumption by getting residents to buy and consume powdered milk. Central to this program was a focus on augmenting livelihoods and purchasing power through subsidized seeds and food and through employment programs. Through these efforts, the nutrition program explicitly linked health to political economy through the household and the food people ate and revealed that a conscious manipulation of what it believed to be the most important aspect of social life would ensure better health. The PCHC treated social life and the biological body together through nutrition. What resulted was a political ecology of health in action.

The Science of Nutrition
and the Economy of Livelihoods

When the PCHC opened its doors in 1940, concerns over malnutrition were beginning to permeate government policy, industry, and the work of important nongovernmental organizations like the South African Institute of Race Relations, which had been so influential for Sidney Kark when he was a student.[6] These concerns came from two different places: First, industry found that malnutrition was negatively affecting its workforce and began to take an interest in nutrition in the Reserves as important for securing productive labor and, by extension, profit. Second, in the 1930s, a number of politicians and activists concerned with the lives of South Africa's poor African population had gained a more prominent voice. Much of their concern centered on nutrition, thanks to the realization that proper (quantifiable) nutrition was key for health.[7] As F. William Fox, a researcher at South Africa's Medical Research Council and foremost expert on "Native" nutrition, wrote, "The importance of diet in relation to health has at last caught the public imagination."[8] These concerns led to efforts to improve diets through health and agricultural education, as the government sought to employ a theory of self-help at the national scale.

Two significant research efforts from the 1930s help explain why there was such a preoccupation with nutrition in the 1940s. First, Kark and Jali's government-sponsored Bantu Nutrition Survey found that malnutrition was a basic condition of life for Africans living in the Reserves. Second, desperate to comprehend why their workers were underperforming, the gold mining industry sponsored a four-hundred-plus-page research report to understand the agricultural and nutritional problems of the areas their workers came from. F. W. Fox and Douglas Back conducted this research in the Ciskei and Transkei Native Reserves directly to the west of Pholela. Like Kark and Jali, Fox and Back found widespread malnutrition. They learned that many of the men recruited from the Reserves to work in the mines were severely malnourished and often ill. These laborers required a period of intensive feeding before they could work at maximum capacity. This, they argued, undermined the labor supply and, by extension, South Africa's economy.[9] On the first page of their report summary they wrote, "Amongst the other factors that go to determine the supply of Native Mine labourers there can be no question that the nutritional background is of fundamental importance; indeed, in the long run it is probably of more importance, though less spectacular than the ravages of tuberculosis, syphilis and malaria, with which of course it is also intimately connected."[10]

These were deeply troubling findings, which growing numbers of doctors, politicians, and activists in South Africa took very seriously. Thanks to these reports, researchers from across South Africa began to realize that the nation's economy was intimately tied to the health and nutrition of the country's poorest people.[11] In South Africa, the profit models of industry had long been premised on the assumption that there was an inexhaustible supply of African workers; therefore, each individual worker was disposable, easily replaced by the next willing recruit.[12] By this logic, white profits would not only be built on the backs of black laborers but would break them. This was racial capitalism in the extreme.

Racial capitalism is a term coined by Cedric Robinson in his book *Black Marxism: The Making of the Black Radical Tradition*. In his book, Robinson rethinks Marx's interpretation of capitalism to argue that it was less a radical break from feudalism and more a continuation of an economic system predicated on differences among groups of people. These differences were racial differences, especially in the context of the Atlantic slave trade. Through his analysis, Robinson argues that race is constitutive of capitalism, which depended on slavery, violence, colonialism, and imperialism in order to thrive.[13] Robin D. G. Kelley explains that "[Robinson] developed [the term 'racial capitalism'] from a description of a *specific* system to a way of understanding the *general* history of modern capitalism."[14] Robinson first encountered the term *racial capitalism* in reference to South Africa's economy under apartheid, where the separation of the races and a racialized labor system were key for profit and capitalist accumulation for whites.[15] This was one of the specifics that led to Robinson's general theory. Walter Rodney's work on Europe's "underdevelopment" of Africa is also instructive for understanding racial capitalism in South Africa. Rodney argues that Europe's success was due to the intentional underdevelopment of Africa, as European profit was predicated on African loss.[16] This was clearly the case in South Africa, where African laborers were considered disposable in order to produce surplus value for whites. And it was this system that underlay concerns over nutrition.

Supported by official state policies, racial capitalism not only affected African workers and industry, but also led to racial segregation and inequality in all aspects of life in South Africa.[17] As Harold Wolpe wrote nearly fifty years ago, industrial capitalism in South Africa was always entangled with racial hierarchies. He writes, "The consequence of this is to integrate race relations with capitalist relations of production to such a degree that the challenge to the one becomes of necessity a challenge to the other."[18] Perhaps ironically, the dependence of all people on the industrial economy for their livelihoods meant that African livelihoods and white livelihoods were inextricably linked. As a result, the low wages that kept rural Africans in poverty while fattening the wallets of whites had consequences for the economy thanks to the inadequate food those wages afforded laborers. Through the bodies of workers, the economies of households in places like Pholela were entangled with the country's biggest industries and the people who profited from them. Therefore, ensuring the long-term health of the economy meant solving the "worker problem," which required an improvement in health and a shift in livelihoods in the Reserves.[19] While in the end these efforts did little to challenge racial capitalism, in the 1930s and 1940s, the government's increasing interest in the lives of Africans showed a recognition that race and economy were co-constituted. It also made the PCHC possible.

Racial capitalism was never limited to South Africa's industries. Until the 1930s, the government and industries had been under the misapprehension that there was enough arable land and enough labor in the Reserves for South Africa's rural, African population to grow the food and livestock they needed to feed themselves. According to this logic, the livelihood practice of subsistence agriculture would underpin the industrial economy, much as it did in places farther north like Nyasaland (present-day Malawi).[20] By the 1930s, however, many officials began to recognize the fallacy of this notion, and by the time Fox and Back's report and the Bantu Nutrition Survey were complete, researchers knew without a doubt that people in the Reserves were not growing, and did not have the land they needed to grow, enough food to feed themselves.[21] As researchers had learned, because residents of these Reserves bought the majority of their calories, the acquisition of a nutritious diet would require both improvements in agriculture *and* improvements in purchasing power (wages).[22] Evidence of this shift in thinking fills archival documents. In these files, it becomes clear that attention shifted from individuals' bad habits to systemic inequities, and from problems in agriculture to a lack of land.[23]

At the same time that South Africa was learning the consequences of its land tenure policies for nutrition, people, and the economy, scientists began to recognize that nutrition was much more complicated than a simple accounting of calories. In the first half of the twentieth century, the period that nutritionist Kenneth Carpenter calls "the golden age of nutrition," scientists isolated the majority of vitamins and minerals important for diets.[24] This was also the period when scientists came to understand the role of nutrients in the body, tying specific diseases like rickets and pellagra to specific nutrients like vitamin D and niacin. And perhaps most important for the story of the PCHC's nutrition program, it was during this period that nutrition science learned that small amounts of nutrients could make a big difference in bodies and in health.[25]

These advances in science provide the backdrop for the intense interest in nutrition in South Africa and the programs and policies that developed from it. Recognizing the importance of nutrition, many policy makers, including the secretary for public health, recommended making foods like dried milk and canned meat available to Africans living in the rural Reserves at a price they could afford.[26] According to the thinking of the day, once rural Africans had enough "protective" foods, they could fill out their diets with easier-to-find and cheaper "supplementary" or "energy yielding" foods like cereals, fats, and sugar for a complete, healthy diet.[27] The individual who consumed this diet would then be a healthy, productive adult, ready to contribute to the economy. In addressing the nutrient deficiencies of Africans specifically, the South African government tacitly acknowledged how entangled the country's political economy was with the racial hierarchy it had imposed.

The more nuanced understanding of nutrition that nutritional science offered combined with economic concerns under racial capitalism to inform official nutritional guidelines. Because government and industry interest in African health and nutrition was tied to concerns about the economy, nutritional recommendations sought to achieve maximum work capacity at minimum cost; the lowest-paid workers (Africans) therefore needed the lowest investment in diet. As a result, nutritional standards, which included basic caloric and micronutrient needs, varied dramatically. For example, guidelines called for 4,500 calories per day for a very active white male, 2,594 for Indian and Coloured families receiving government relief, and 1,827 for an African family living in Johannesburg.[28] In addition, recommendations for certain aspects of diets like animal protein varied from thirty-five grams per day for a white male to zero grams per day for an African family, or vitamin C at thirty-seven milligrams for an African family and eight milligrams for an Indian or Coloured family. The breakdown of individual needs in standards like these had wide-ranging implications, as these recommendations helped set the regulation of food rations in the mines and helped form the basis of policies from price setting to health and agricultural reform to school meal and other feeding schemes.[29] Through these and other official recommendations, nutritional science was enrolled in a national politics of inequality.

In some ways, these race-specific nutrition guidelines broke from the nutritional science of the time, which saw bodies as interchangeable, interacting with individual nutrients in predictable ways. In others, it fit well with a science that was just beginning to produce the kinds of guidelines that were the precursors to the nutritional information disaggregated by age and gender that we encounter today on food packages.[30] In South Africa, in practice, nutrition science was always shaped by race, which was, of course, correlated with poverty. For the South African state, racial difference was central to its understanding of social life as it applied to nutrition and health more generally. In her book *Starving on a Full Stomach*, Diana Wylie argues that just as industrial capitalism restructured landscapes and livelihoods, it also shaped the production and application of scientific knowledge, including nutritional science.[31] For Wylie, the science of nutrition was always shaped by the race-based social stratification that had long underpinned the economy and social life in South Africa. She argues that progressive scientists were as focused on race as conservative scientists, but they articulated it differently. For these scientists, the failure of African nutrition was a failure of culture, rather than an inherent inferiority of the African body. Africans made "poor choices," because their approach to food was "unscientific." The end result was ill health. As Wylie writes, nutritional and health "progress would be limited, not by their bodies, but by their resistance to the lessons of modern science."[32] By this logic, malnutrition and ill health were still the fault of Africans, even if not problems of biological difference.

The solution on display in Pholela was to educate Africans in nutritional science and to encourage them to make better choices—to help people help themselves. This was the kind of paternalism that marked progressive politics in South Africa as it mixed with the industrial economy and racial capitalism. By the logic of the day, to be good citizens, to contribute to the economy, Africans would choose nutritious food, thereby ensuring that they would have healthy bodies, which would help keep the economy going.[33] Overall, the result was a nutrition science in practice that distinguished by race in such a way that Africans were always at the bottom of a hierarchy as either not needing as many calories and nutrients as people of other races or as making poor and unscientific choices.[34]

Confronting Malnutrition and Ill Health in Pholela

Troubled, if not surprised, by what they found when they first came to Pholela, the Karks and their staff began a nutrition program almost immediately in an effort to use the latest in nutritional science to improve the lives of residents. Combining health education with new foods, this program started in the clinic and soon moved to the communities of the Designated Area. The health center quickly settled on a two-part program focused on vegetable production at home (to increase micronutrients) and the purchase of powdered milk (to increase macronutrients). The PCHC designed this program to combine women's agricultural labor and men's wages earned working away from home to improve nutrition, and by extension, health. For the Karks, nutritional deficiencies and needs were first and foremost related to poverty. By this logic, malnutrition was a social problem where social life was understood through racial capitalism. In developing its nutrition program, the PCHC sought to combine attention to the social context of lives and livelihoods and to the biology of bodies in order to improve health. In so doing, the health center believed that the nutrition program would demonstrate that social medicine was the key to improving health in Pholela and beyond.

Overcoming Micronutrient Shortfalls:
The "Grow and Eat More Vegetables" Campaign

The PCHC's "Grow and Eat More Vegetables" campaign began with the establishment of a demonstration garden on the grounds of the health center. Covering an acre, the garden's lush green plants and bright red, green, and yellow vegetables offered a verdant oasis. Upon closer look, the contents of the garden were unfamiliar to most residents. In this space, the staff experimented with a variety of vegetables, filling this acre of health center land with new foods like cabbage, spinach, carrots, tomatoes, sweet potatoes, peppers, and beetroot.[35] Not all vegetables grew equally well, however, as Pholela's environment and climate determined what would thrive.[36] To enhance the garden's productivity, staff fertilized it with compost produced in the health center's model compost pit. They also built a very basic irrigation scheme to ensure that the garden had plenty of water during dry periods. Unlike home gardens where residents planted maize, beans, pumpkins, and greens all together in what health center staff saw as a haphazard mess, the vegetables in the clinic's demonstration garden were planted in rows in distinct beds, with carrots in one section, maize in another, and beans in yet another. Staff separated these beds with narrow rows of hard-packed, brown dirt, giving the garden a checkerboard-like aesthetic.

The health center staff planted fruits and vegetables based first and foremost on their knowledge of nutrient content, as the garden became a landscape for health. Beds of carrots became compartments of beta-carotene and vitamin A, and the lemon trees that lined the garden's perimeter ringed its matrix with vitamin C. Thanks to the nutritional logics that underpinned its layout, the demonstration garden came to be the place to assemble the building blocks for basic nutrition, and by extension, for health; it provided the blueprint for a healthy family. In addition, this clear layout taught residents what these new vegetables looked like at every stage of growth, and hands-on lessons with health assistants in the garden taught residents techniques for managing those crops while they grew. With just a quick look, one could easily see what a carrot looked like when it was growing or what a cabbage looked like when it was ready to be picked. When combined with lessons about the value of nutrition for health, the garden was quite literally the landscape of social medicine.

Seeds and science were not enough. To ensure that vegetables grew, the health center needed people to plant, weed, tend, and harvest them. In other words, the garden required labor to thrive. At the health center's demonstration garden, any and every member of the staff from the doctors to the cleaners could be seen tending crops. Health center staff encouraged patients who attended the clinic, especially those who came for special programs like the mother and child wellness program, to work in the demonstration garden.[37] This collaborative arrangement provided a hands-on training ground where health center staff taught area residents the nuts and bolts of both agricultural and nutritional science in the very space that had been built to join them; in return, the health center received the help it needed to keep the garden going. Patients and others who helped in the garden took home parcels of fresh vegetables and seeds on occasion. The parcels promoted good health, as these new, micronutrient-packed vegetables found their way into residents' gardens, cooking pots, bellies, and the cells that made up their bodies. Health center staff believed that once patients had knowledge about nutrition and agricultural best practices and the skills to implement them, they would plant their own vegetable gardens, sowing nutrients into the soil of their homestead landscapes and integrating them into their diets.[38] In so doing, residents would take charge of improving their own health right at home.

Those patients and health center visitors who worked in the garden were not the only people to receive parcels of food. Once the vegetables had reached maturity, health center staff harvested them and the doctors gave out prescriptions of vegetables from the demonstration garden, thereby integrating the garden directly into medical aspects of health center practice. The doctors saw these prescriptions as the most important medications for nutrition-related illnesses, malnutrition, and general ill health. The demonstration garden's scientific logic and organization allowed a doctor to quickly choose a cluster of micronutrients best matched to the needs of his or her patient.[39] The doctor could then take their patient outside and show them where in the soil of the garden landscape these important building blocks for health grew. Pointing to a patch of green peas, for example, the doctors would explain that this niacin-rich food was key for treating and preventing pellagra. After lessons in the garden and the doctor's office about the "value in health" of the vegetables, patients went to the pharmacy counter, turned in their prescription, and collected a packet of vegetables, just as they collected other medications.[40] Through the garden and the pharmacy, the health center integrated vegetables seamlessly into the clinic's treatment regime, as agricultural, nutritional, and biomedical sciences came together to improve the health of residents.

The PCHC did not stop at food prescriptions; to help ensure that these newly grown and prescribed nutrients made their way into residents' bodies, health center staff taught area residents how to prepare their new vegetables in ways that preserved their nutrients. Residents recall that these lessons taught them to wash their vegetables before cooking, to lightly boil rather than fry, and to reserve nutrient-rich vegetable water for cooking maize meal. The health center staff reasoned that by learning and implementing new cooking techniques, residents would reap maximum health benefit from the new food they would be consuming. And as the story of Gogo Ngcobo's garden from the introduction reveals, these lessons lasted.

The health center's efforts to change agricultural and cooking practices soon expanded beyond the clinic grounds into the communities that made up the Designated Area. In these places, the health center staff established demonstration gardens at schools and key households. These gardens became satellite sites, offering spaces closer to home for area residents, including schoolchildren, to learn about gardening and nutrition and to practice new techniques. This was especially useful for those who did not attend the clinic regularly. The local school lunch programs, supported through a countrywide nutrition effort and run by the health center, used vegetables from school gardens to supplement the store-bought food purchased for daily meals.[41] The gardens were therefore important for two reasons: they provided lessons in gardening and nutrition to schoolchildren and their parents, and they provided nutrients to children who were at a crucial point in their cognitive and physical development. Pholela's doctors saw these daily nutritious meals as especially important in light of their discovery of the large extent of seasonal malnutrition among schoolchildren and the long-term health implications of that malnutrition.[42]

Health center staff understood that in order for the "Grow and Eat More Vegetables" campaign to succeed over the long term, the vegetables that the health center promoted needed to be integrated into the home production of area residents. In other words, the health center needed to shift the subsistence agriculture portion of residents' livelihood strategies. Once the health center's demonstration gardens at the clinic and at area schools had proven successful, it used the health assistants to expand the "Grow and Eat More Vegetables" campaign to every Designated Area homestead that was willing to participate. In so doing, it integrated its nutrition program into its broader efforts to remake homesteads.[43]

The results of the home garden program speak for themselves. Within the first ten years of the PCHC's establishment, the proportion of homes with summer gardens in the Designated Area went from 64.8 percent to 88.8 percent. And between 1941 and 1951 the percentage of households with winter gardens, which are particularly important for seasonal malnutrition, went from 54.3 percent to 69 percent.[44] More importantly, during the initial survey in 1941, the health center found that residents planted only six different crops in vegetable gardens, most of which were the same as the crops planted in fields. By 1950, there were twenty-five varieties of vegetables,[45] and by 1951, there were thirty-three.[46] This increase in crop diversity had a dramatic impact on diets, eating habits, and health. By the late 1950s, it would have been hard to imagine a diet that did not include beetroot, lemons, and carrots (and the micronutrients they contained), all of which were virtually unknown before the arrival of the Karks and their staff. This shift in garden contents helped to ensure that residents had a wider supply of the various micronutrients they needed for a healthy, balanced diet, while the increase in winter gardens helped ensure that those micronutrients lasted into the winter and spring.

Health center efforts to improve access to micronutrients extended beyond the homestead garden too. During harvest season, the PCHC staff organized a weekly market at the health center where people could buy and sell excess produce.[47] Over time, the markets became so popular that residents held them daily at the health center and weekly in various locations throughout the Designated Area.[48] These vegetable markets were particularly important for families who had small or unproductive gardens. At the markets, they could purchase fresh vegetables to supplement their home production and the maize meal they bought at the store, thereby increasing the nutrients they consumed. In rare cases, these markets allowed families with particularly productive gardens to earn all of the money they needed to support themselves. This meant that the men who had migrated for work could return home without jeopardizing their family's livelihood. Once the men returned, the family would have more labor with which to produce more food in order to earn more money from their home gardens. For example, the third medical director of the PCHC, Cecil Slome, recounted the story of one woman, "Mrs. H," whose garden was so prolific that she actually earned more than her husband, who worked as a migrant laborer in town. As a result, when he returned home to receive treatment for an aortic aneurysm, his wife could support him, and he did not need to return to work. And when he passed away, Mrs. H was able to continue to support the family from her home garden, and therefore she did not have to move to the city, leaving her children to make do without her. According to Slome, had she not received lessons and seeds from the health center, had there been no demand for vegetables in the community, and had she not had a market through which to sell her produce—had the health center's nutrition program never come to Pholela—her family would have been destitute when her husband got sick.[49]

In many senses, the "Grow and Eat More Vegetables" campaign exemplified social medicine in Pholela. It sought to alter the subsistence agriculture component of household livelihood practices to improve health in the context of racial capitalism. It linked food, which was a key product of these livelihood practices, to medicine and health through prescriptions and lessons about nutrition. And it took place at the clinic, in communities, and at people's homes. This was social medicine in action. It was also remarkably successful. As the micronutrients in diets increased, health improved. In the first ten years of health center practice, the number of patients seeking treatment for illnesses related to malnutrition dropped from more than eight cases a month to fewer than eight a year. At the same time, infant and crude mortality plummeted, and new cases of infectious diseases dropped.[50] While neither new infection rates nor mortality rates were directly related to nutrition, the indirect relationships were significant, as changes in gardens led to changes in bodies.

In its efforts to give Pholela's residents the building blocks for good health through better nutrition, the PCHC soon expanded its nutrition program to include a focus on the macronutrient protein. While this made sense in terms of the specific nutrition-related illnesses in Pholela, it was also very prescient, anticipating what would become the preoccupation of many nutrition-related international development projects later in the century.[51] As the health center began to work on increasing protein consumption, it quickly discovered that this aspect of the nutrition program would be more difficult than the vegetable program. There was little protein available locally and there were consumption restrictions on what was available. As a result, in addition to changing people's subsistence agricultural practices, the health center realized it would need to augment purchasing habits and purchasing power. In other words, if the health center was to increase protein consumption, it needed to intervene in the political economy of the household.

While protein can come from certain nuts and legumes, its most common source in Pholela was animals. And yet people owned very little livestock and taboos limited the consumption of the livestock protein available. The result was very little protein in diets when the PCHC began its work in 1940. Take the example of eggs. Rich in protein, eggs supply all the essential amino acids people need, as well as vitamins A and B$_{12}$ and riboflavin, choline, and phosphorus.[52] Because there were quite a few chickens in Pholela, the health center reasoned that changing egg consumption patterns would provide a relatively quick fix to nutrition problems. As a result, early in the PCHC's health extension program, health assistants visited homesteads to teach women how to cook eggs and about the importance of the protein inside them. In particular, they focused on cooking eggs for infants in order to ensure that they would receive protein at this critical point in their development.[53]

In spite of these efforts, however, progress was slow. As residents explain, people believed that eating eggs was like "stealing from the next generation," because each egg had the potential to become a chicken. In addition, dogs ate many of the eggs that chickens laid because nests were not protected. These two factors meant that residents of any age rarely consumed the eggs their chickens laid. Once the health center realized these barriers, staff members helped residents build chicken coops to protect eggs from dogs and explained the importance of eggs for the next generation. With these efforts, eggs became relatively common in the diets of infants and children, as children consumed eggs on average three to four times a week during the more productive season. But even this ready source of protein was limited by the number of chickens each family could afford to keep. As a result, adults ate eggs only rarely, until stores began to stock them and families began buying them.[54]

Because eggs could not fully address the problem of protein in diets, the health center sought to increase milk consumption. This was different from the start, as milk was entangled with both national political-economic forces and familial social relationships through food taboos. Health center staff began their effort to increase consumption by focusing on children and young women and on the livestock already in Pholela. These efforts were quickly stymied. Soon after their arrival, the Karks found that there were very few cows in Pholela and that those cows that were present belonged to very few families. Less than half of all households had even a single cow that produced milk in the summer, the height of the milking season.[55] Without enough cows, there was not enough protein-filled milk or *amasi* (a liquid, yogurt-like food that was the most common way to consume cow's milk) for any but the wealthiest residents.[56] This had tremendous health implications. Rich in protein, cow's milk is also a good source of calcium, potassium, niacin, riboflavin, and vitamins A, C, D, K, and E, making it the kind of highly nutritious food the health center was looking for to combat malnutrition and shore up baseline health. The uneven distribution and the sheer lack of cows meant that Pholela's residents would need to find this nutrition elsewhere.

As if scarcity was not enough, health center efforts to increase the consumption of the small amount of fresh milk available from area cows met even more resistance than efforts to increase egg consumption. In Pholela, newly married women followed *hlonipha* customs, which prohibited the consumption of milk and amasi in their new homes while their husbands' ancestors got to know and recognize them. If these women did not follow these customs, they might not be protected from ill health by their new ancestors; in other words, the health-related consequences of not following hlonipha-related milk consumption prohibitions were dire. When the PCHC taught lessons about the importance of milk consumption, they found that very few women were willing to risk the protection of new ancestors for an increase in protein in their diets. In early annual reports and in publications, health center staff often complained about this, writing about the "backwardness" of Pholela's residents.[57] As the second medical director of the PCHC, Dr. John Cassel, wrote, "Whatever the underlying reasons, it soon became evident that the taking of milk by girls and especially by married women had a powerful emotional connotation. In the face of those deep-seated beliefs, no mere conviction of the nutritional value of milk could be expected to change the practice."[58] The cultural racism that Wylie writes about in terms of the application of scientific knowledge was clearly at work in the PCHC's nutrition program.

As the health center grappled with the problem of hlonipha and the limited supply of local fresh milk, it began to supply milk powder to patients suffering from malnutrition and related illnesses in the very same food prescriptions that included vegetables from the demonstration garden.[59] Soon after their incorporation into prescriptions, these milk powder rations were integrated into many health center programs, like its well-child program. Participants soon received supplies as a part of their weekly visit to the health center. But as the "Grow and Eat More Vegetables" program revealed, if the health center was to really improve health over the long term, it would need to change what people produced and procured at home. Recognizing that Pholela's residents got the bulk of their calories and food from the store, the PCHC staff knew that they would need to change purchasing habits. Milk became a key food through which to do just that. Once residents had begun to consume powdered milk from the health center, the PCHC arranged for a local white farmer to sell fresh milk to Pholela's residents, and it encouraged local shops to stock milk powder. Much to its surprise and delight, there was quickly great demand, as people began to regularly purchase both fresh and powdered milk.[60] As in the case of new vegetables, integrating milk powder into residents' diets first through prescriptions accompanied by education helped to ensure that milk would find a permanent place in the diets and bodies of residents.

By turning to purchased milk as opposed to milk from residents' cows, the health center overcame the limits of local livestock and the range it subsisted on, all of which were constrained by the limited land and labor available; it overcame one key aspect of racial capitalism.[61] In addition, purchased milk was not subject to the same hlonipha restrictions. This was because milk-related taboos were not directed toward milk in general, but rather toward milk from the livestock of a woman's new family. Those livestock were the conduit to her new ancestors, and therefore key for ensuring good health. As a result, women could consume protein-packed milk powder without fear that it might affect their absorption into their new family line and the health-related protection that it afforded them.[62] They could "protect" their nutrient-related health, to borrow a term from the nutrition pamphlets of the day, without making themselves vulnerable to other illnesses.

Because store-bought and powdered milk sat outside the social relations of the family, it was quickly a food everyone consumed on a daily basis, especially in households that did not produce fresh amasi.[63] For young women and children, it would be hard to overestimate the importance of this shift, because for the first time they had equal access to protein. And just as in the case of micronutrients, when protein was added to the diets of pregnant and lactating women and children, the long-term health-related results were impressive. Between 1950 and 1953, the rates of kwashiorkor among infants decreased from 14.85 per 1,000 to 3.29 per 1,000, and milder forms of protein deficiency in children also dropped markedly.[64] While remarkable for its immediate impact, this reduction in malnutrition had even more impressive effects in the longer term, as children sustained healthier growth rates and improved cognitive development and as healthy children grew into healthy adults. Thanks to an overall increase in protein consumption, the impact of the PCHC would be felt for years.

But simply ensuring that milk powder was available for purchase did not necessarily guarantee it a place in the regular diet of residents over the long term. After all, milk powder was more expensive than maize meal, and many residents were on a very tight budget. While the provision of milk powder for health through prescriptions helped erase economic barriers to good nutrition at first, without employment for Pholela's poorest people, those divisions would return once the responsibility for acquiring protein shifted to residents. To ameliorate these differences in access, the PCHC set out to employ as many local residents from as many different households as possible. It reasoned that if people had an income with which to buy powdered milk, they would.[65]

As the health center expanded, so too did its need for staff, and by the mid-1940s it was one of, if not the biggest, employer in the area. From health assistants to lab assistants, from cleaners to cooks, there were lots of jobs with varying skill requirements. People employed by the clinic took home leftover milk powder and extra vegetables, and they could transplant seedlings from the demonstration garden and collect leftover seeds for their home gardens. As a result, their formal connection to the clinic helped them informally. Residents recall that employees had particularly diverse and productive vegetable gardens and their incomes enabled them to buy more milk powder. In addition, many women took advantage of new, less formal opportunities for employment that resulted from the PCHC. For example, health center doctors and nurses employed residents as domestic servants, a handful of residents set up informal stands to sell food to people attending the health center, and still others made a living through local produce markets as the employment impact of the PCHC exceeded the boundaries of its work. This new local employment, which focused on spreading resources across the population, shifted the local political economy, evening out disparities. As an added benefit, by providing employment close to home, the PCHC ensured that there was more labor to work the fields and tend gardens at the end of the workday. As a result, this large-scale employment effort had implications for both aspects of livelihood practices.

PCHC employment was particularly beneficial to those women who otherwise would be dependent on wages from men who worked at distant locations. While they might have to wait months between remittances from male family members, local employment meant regular infusions of cash into households. This regularity allowed for more consistent shopping and often for the purchase of perishable foods in local markets. This was particularly important in the hungry spring months when families could purchase fresh food to overcome seasonal nutrient shortfalls. In addition, as older women explain today, as women increasingly earned money, they made more of the purchasing decisions.[66] Thanks in part to the fact that so many of them were involved with the health center, their purchasing patterns began to follow the lessons they were learning about food and nutrition as they bought more and more milk and milk powder, thereby increasing household protein consumption.

By promoting the conditions for widespread employment, the PCHC changed residents', and especially women's, expectations about work, where food should come from, how it should be procured, and who should decide. Residents explained that as time progressed, milk powder became something they regularly purchased from the shop, not simply because it made their family healthier, but also because they liked it and they couldn't imagine their tea or their morning porridge without it. In changing access, knowledge, and taste—in intervening in the social world—the PCHC guaranteed that the majority of people in Pholela would consume protein regularly. This protein put an end to acute malnutrition and helped boost people's immune systems to prevent other illnesses. By 1950, kwashiorkor had essentially disappeared. In the PCHC's elegant solution to malnutrition and illness more generally, the social and the medical aspects of the health center's social medicine came together.

A Political Ecology of Nutrition in Pholela

As its most important and far-reaching scheme, the PCHC's nutrition program formed the bedrock of its social medicine practice. Significantly, it focused on food, rather than pharmaceuticals or other therapeutics, as its key treatment and as preventive medicine. Grown in Pholela's landscape, the new micronutrient-packed vegetables tied improvements in the health of the individual and the family to the homestead. Thanks to the PCHC, residents planted seeds purchased at a distance and learned scientific agricultural techniques perfected in research centers in South Africa and as far away as the United States. They did this to maximize yields of nutritious food with the belief that those nutrients would make for healthier bodies. Even before the PCHC went to work, the homestead landscape was indelibly linked to the industrial centers of South Africa through labor. But through these new vegetables and new techniques, Pholela's homestead garden landscapes formed new connections with the rest of South Africa and beyond. At the same time, changes in spending patterns, particularly in terms of the purchase of powdered milk, linked other improvements in health to cash wages earned at home and away and to South Africa's industrial agricultural sector. Together, these new foods had a dramatic impact on residents' health as malnutrition all but disappeared.

The PCHC staff was successful in part because they recognized that Pholela's landscape and its residents were part of a much broader political economy. When the Karks arrived in Pholela, they already understood that what today we call racial capitalism played a role in the nutrition and health of residents. As they saw it, a racist set of policies embedded in the needs of the industrial economy had left Pholela's residents poor, malnourished, and unhealthy; this was the social life that underpinned social medicine for the health center. What the Karks and their team had not yet realized was the role that the political economy played in what land was available to residents and what impact it had on the food they could produce. It was this realization that led the PCHC to develop a nutrition program that augmented purchasing power and worked to change spending habits while improving agricultural output. Through this program, the PCHC came to recognize that the landscapes that affected residents' health were much larger than those of Pholela's communities and homesteads.

To understand the possibilities and limitations of the PCHC's nutrition program, I offer a political ecology that combines scholarship that examines the relationships between political economy and health with scholarship that details the role of livelihoods in shaping environmental and natural resource management. First, to understand the relationships between large-scale political-economic forces and the uneven health of individuals, a number of medical anthropologists offer the concept of structural violence. This concept connotes the impact of poverty and inequality on the health of the world's poor.[67] For example, through cases like basic malnutrition, diarrheal diseases, state violence, and infectious diseases like HIV/AIDS, Paul Farmer details how political agreements and international trade and aid harm disempowered individuals in Haiti. In this analysis, the global scale interacts with the individual scale to lead to illness and death through the state. The rampant malnutrition and ill health that the health center team found when it arrived in Pholela is an example of structural violence. Second, political ecologists have long been interested in the role of livelihoods in shaping environments and people, recognizing that individual and household livelihoods are shaped by broader political-economic forces.[68] Bringing these two approaches together connects large-scale structures like racial capitalism in South Africa with household- and individual-scale political economies and with bodies. The subfield of political ecologies of health does this explicitly, recognizing the body as a site for examining the interactions of large-scale political-economic forces and more local socionatural environments.[69] In this framing, bodies are always simultaneously social and biological, and so is human health.[70]

In many senses, the PCHC's program did exactly what political ecology calls on practitioners to do. For example, in their early work, *Land Degradation and Society*, Piers Blaikie and Harold Brookfield demonstrate that soil erosion is not simply the result of poor land use practices employed by peasants. Rather, erosion is the result of limited land and labor (political economy) and the particularities of soil, topography, and vegetation (ecology); it was the result of human–nonhuman relationships. Through this analysis, they shift the blame for erosion from the actions of local people to the specific combination of the environment in which those people live and the multiscalar political economy in which they labor.[71] This approach teaches much about the entanglements of soil and people, water and economies, mountain slopes and labor; it teaches much about the relationships between land degradation and society. This type of approach, which combines an attention to the biophysical environment (nonhumans) and an attention to social structures (humans), is exactly that which guided the work of the PCHC. As a program anchored in the ecology of Pholela's homesteads and the political economy of South Africa, the PCHC's nutrition program was political ecology realized, some forty years before the work of Blaikie and Brookfield.[72]

Addressing malnutrition also requires an attention to people's bodies and the cells they are made of. In other words, a political ecology of health requires a scaling down to individual bodies where the nutrients in the beetroot and carrots residents grew and the powdered milk they purchased helped to ensure that their cells functioned as they should, that they grew well, that they had good vision, and that they could fight off the infectious diseases that they came into contact with. As the impressive statistics of the health center reveal, these nutrients shifted residents' "internal ecologies" for the better.[73] Through nutrition, the large national scale and the microscopic sub-bodily scale (and all of the scales in between) combined to produce healthier people.[74] In this analysis, causality is clear. It follows the scalar logic of nutritional and biomedical sciences: increases in nutrients lead to predictable changes in cellular structures, which lead to healthy growth, improvements in immune system function, and so on. Likewise, the political economy acted across scales in ways that social scientists expect: discriminatory landownership policies based on race and an industrial economy with an insatiable need for cheap African labor combined to circumscribe livelihood possibilities for residents, thereby negatively affecting their nutrition and health. By bringing these two causal chains together, a political ecology of health links what is happening inside of people's bodies with their gardens and with the political system that determines land tenure and the economic forces that determine who can work where and when. This scalar logic also emerged from the PCHC's early mapping and surveying efforts. The health center understood these relationships and utilized the lessons of nutritional and biomedical science on the one hand and the social sciences on the other to improve health.

The health center's nutrition program highlights the efficacy of its understanding of social life for its efforts to fight malnutrition. As it sought to improve nutrition through subsistence agriculture and purchased food, the staff of the PCHC accepted and embraced the mixed livelihood reality of Pholela. It did so because it saw people's health as embedded in social relationships and as read through the political economy of livelihoods. By focusing on livelihoods, the PCHC avoided conflicts with other aspects of social life, like those that manifest in hlonipha restrictions. In embracing a vision of social life rooted in political economy, which recognized the importance of wage labor through large-scale employment efforts and encouraged the consumption of particular store-bought foods, the health center acknowledged the ways in which nutrition-related health was linked to racial capitalism in South Africa. This made its nutrition program a decidedly social intervention.[75]

Through its nutrition program, the PCHC succeeded in ameliorating some of the most pernicious aspects of poverty and inequality, even though it never managed to erase economic difference completely. One of the greatest ironies of the nutrition program, however, and one which a detailed political-ecology analysis reveals, was that the program produced new nutrition- and health-related dependencies on national and global markets that would eventually undermine its success. For example, for the people of Pholela to continue consuming the protein in powdered milk, companies would need to continue to manufacture it; households would need to have enough cash to buy it; and shop owners would need to find selling it profitable enough to keep it in stock. Just as other forces beyond residents' control like weather and pests shaped how much they could produce at home, the government's regulatory body, the labor needs of South Africa's industries, and the movements of regional and global markets shaped how much they could buy. As a result, as the PCHC catalyzed new relationships between the broader political economy, Pholela's homesteads, and the bodies of individuals, it also produced new vulnerabilities.[76] While the health center was working in Pholela, residents remained somewhat protected from these fluctuations. If powdered milk became too expensive for families to buy and people were in danger of malnutrition, the health center might increase prescriptions or it might negotiate a lower price with area shops to ensure that the powdered milk still found its way into people's diets. In other words, the health center's presence in the context of health and market forces mediated the effects of racial capitalism on residents' diets and health.[77] But once the government seriously curtailed the PCHC's services in the early 1960s, residents no longer had these protections, leaving them and their health more vulnerable to fluctuations in price and income over which they had no control.

As a result, and as residents explained, their health suffered. The tenuous links between the cells in their bodies and South Africa's brand of racial capitalism through food and nutrients were easily unsettled once health center operations were curtailed. As scholars remind us, people living in poverty, like Pholela's residents, take on the burdens of their precarious lives in the cells of their bodies.[78] By augmenting livelihood practices to improve nutrition, the health center intervened in the very place where, in the words of Karen Barad, the "large-scale organization of power" linked up with "local practices" in order to improve the health of the body.[79] The PCHC recognized that livelihoods are and always have been embodied, and that therefore, the health of residents was the embodiment of South Africa's changing political economy. This was emblematic of the health center's understanding of social life through a lens of racial capitalism as well as a program that included nonhumans in an effort to improve health by shaping social life. Herein lies one of the limitations of the social medicine practiced in Pholela. No matter how much the health center taught Pholela's residents and no matter how great an effort the staff made to change their behavior, without large-scale poverty relief, changes would only be temporary. With at least some of the roots of ill health firmly planted in the racist policies of the minority government and the needs of the industrial economy, the results of the social medicine practiced in Pholela would never be as radical as its practitioners hoped.[80]

In early 2008, when I began my long fieldwork period, global food prices were skyrocketing and the price of food was a topic on everyone's mind. By then, households relied almost entirely on store-bought food for their day-to-day needs. As prices increased and money got tighter, people would spend less on foods that seemed like luxuries—meat, fresh milk, amasi, fresh vegetables, and even powdered milk, reserving their limited cash for basics like maize meal, bread, and cooking oil, which together supplied sufficient calories, if not nutrients. As I spoke with Pholela's residents about the global food crisis, it became clear that this kind of purchasing triage was not new. It also became clear that many of them anticipated consequences for their health. Thanks in part to the PCHC and its health education, they knew that nutrition was important and that they thought that they had a responsibility to buy nutritious food to have a healthy family. And yet, just as would be the case in the 1960s, in 2008 residents could do little with their knowledge of nutrition; they were at the mercy of racial capitalism.

4

Witchcraft and the Limits of Social Medicine

Wrapped in a sweater, I sat under the fluo-
rescent lights in the overly air-conditioned National Archives of South Africa
reading through the yellowing pages of the PCHC annual reports. I was im-
pressed by the evidence of health improvements and homestead transformations that filled the pages. But alongside rapidly increasing numbers of household gardens and decreasing cases of syphilis were two numbers that weren't
changing: cases of tuberculosis infections and pit latrine installation in homesteads. As I read the annual reports, it became clear that in spite of intensive
health education and other efforts, the health center's program was not universally successful. Indeed, nine years into the efforts to establish pit latrines, just
3 percent of the households in the Designated Area had them; seven years after
that, the number had climbed to only 8 percent.[1] The statistics for TB were similarly unimpressive.

What was not clear from the annual reports but became clearer as I began
to understand health and healing from Pholela was why these programs had
failed. Take the example of pit latrines. The PCHC's inability to get residents to
build pit latrines, which were integral to its waste-disposal plan, had much to
do with residents' efforts to prevent witchcraft illness in Pholela. An *umthakathi*
could make a person sick through her feces, but to do so, she needed to know
where it was. Therefore, to stay healthy, it was important to hide where people
defecated. Pit latrines did the opposite, exposing people and making them vulnerable to a witchcraft illness. For residents, the risks of contracting witchcraft
illness by centralizing and containing human waste outweighed the benefits of
separating bacteria from feces.

In Pholela, residents have long suffered and continue to suffer from witchcraft illnesses. As the PCHC saw it, witchcraft illnesses were cultural explana-

tions for biomedical diseases. As such, they were evidence of "backward beliefs." The health center staff's choice of the word belief is significant. A subtle insult, articulating residents' attention to illness beyond the purview of social medicine as belief showed disdain for and frustration at what appeared to them to be a contempt for education and an unwillingness to accept the lessons of science. For Pholela's residents, however, witchcraft posed a very real threat to their bodily well-being. Moreover, witchcraft illnesses were never biomedical illnesses by a different name (illnesses that just happened, in the local taxonomy); they were entirely distinct, caused by something else. As residents and healers explain, witchcraft illnesses are always the result of uneasy relationships among people, things, and harder-to-categorize beings like ancestors and incantations. Unpacking the specifics of what causes witchcraft illnesses and how they are treated offers an understanding of health as more-than-human entanglement.

Recognizing health as more-than-human entanglement opens up the questions of what makes people sick and what constitutes social life. It also makes clear the limits of a social medicine practice that understands social life through political economy and the social sciences and a practice that relies in part on (social) relationships that include nonhuman things. The PCHC's inability to address, understand, accept, and even see witchcraft illness became a barrier to the full-scale success it sought. While the lack of pit latrines offers one example, this failure was most obvious and most serious in the failure of the PCHC's antituberculosis campaign, its most unsuccessful program.

To understand the lessons of witchcraft illnesses, in this chapter, I examine TB alongside the witchcraft illness *idliso*, which have overlapping symptoms. This symmetrical analysis has a long history in science studies.[2] As Stacey Langwick explains, "The symmetry principle [in science studies] suggests that all assertions of truth or fact, whether they are judged to be rational or irrational, accurate or inaccurate, possible or impossible, should be approached by [scholars] in the same way."[3] For science studies scholars, this means applying the same analytical rigor (of social systems) to the claims of science as to those of other knowledge systems. This approach enables an analysis of illness that is not comparative, but parallel. Analyzing TB and idliso in parallel as two illnesses affecting people challenges scientific models of causality, offering an understanding of health and illness rooted in relationships and read through entanglements; it therefore offers a different, more expansive vision of health and of social life.

A Note on Witchcraft

Scholars of Africa have long been interested in questions of witchcraft. For those versed in this scholarship, the approach I offer here is quite different. As a result, it is worth quickly examining this literature to make my point of departure clear. As many scholars have noted, witchcraft in Africa has long played an important role in regulating social life.[4] In this sense, the power of *abathakathi* (plural of umthakathi) over day-to-day life extended well beyond the *imithi* (plural of *umuthi*) they produce to the social life of the community. With the onset of the colonial state and the rise of missionaries, witchcraft became a crime, as did making accusations of witchcraft. The state understood witchcraft as a way to articulate power battles through a sphere that was beyond its control. This was, at least in part, true, as the very possibility of witchcraft in communities played an important role in regulating behavior. But with the incorporation of witchcraft into colonial law, Africans' concerns with witchcraft became about both relationships with family members and neighbors and relations with the state. The possibility of state sanction often kept fights between families and neighbors from getting too serious, as everyone sought to protect their bodily health, social relationships, and relationship to the colonial state.

Scholars have argued that in many instances, these efforts to regulate witchcraft through the legal system forced its practices underground, enhancing the perception that witchcraft is a clandestine activity. Adam Ashforth expands on this understanding to examine politics in postapartheid South Africa, arguing that the state's changing stance on witchcraft became one site of insecurity for the country's disenfranchised population. In this analysis, concerns with changes in sociopolitical forces are articulated and experienced through what Ashforth terms "spiritual insecurity," or concerns over witchcraft.[5] There are parallels here with the PCHC's articulation of social life through political economy. This and other analyses are important for understanding the ways in which witchcraft is imbricated in social structures in communities as well as colonial and minority-rule state projects. But the relegation of witchcraft to the realm of human-only social life makes it hard to understand the symptoms ill people suffer from; it makes it hard to recognize that witchcraft causes physical illness. The result is that both the biomedical and the social sciences understand witchcraft to be something separate from the processes that cause a cough or a sore back; both see witchcraft as separate from biological health. Like the colonial state, scholars of both biomedicine and the social sciences see witchcraft as that which lies beyond medicine and science more generally.[6] But as the PCHC's nutrition and homestead programs reveal, social life is never divorced from material life. In this book, and in this chapter specifically, I recognize health as emerging from the relationships embedded in social life, where that social life includes humans, nonhumans, and harder-to-categorize beings. As the people whose stories I offer demonstrate, witchcraft makes people physically ill; the manifestation of the social relations is physical. In this framework, social life includes physical beings as well as people, structures, and beings and forces often relegated to the realm of the occult.

I posit that understanding health and healing from Pholela requires an understanding that Pholela's residents suffer and suffered from witchcraft illnesses including idliso—real, physical illnesses, and not mere translations of more familiar illnesses like tuberculosis. Recognizing witchcraft illness as physical illness is a difficult leap, and one that contrasts with much of the scholarship about witchcraft and traditional healing more generally. There is much to be learned by accepting, as a provocation at the very least, that people suffer physical illness as a result of witchcraft and then examining how and why witchcraft works. In the pages that follow, I take up this provocation to rethink health, causality, and social life from Pholela.

Idliso, Tuberculosis, and the Limits of Health Center Practice

By 1952, just twelve years after the PCHC was founded, many indicators showed that it was a rousing success. Yet tuberculosis rates for both continuing cases and new infections continued to climb. This was in spite of the fact that throughout the 1940s and 1950s, the PCHC invested heavily in and implemented a large-scale TB eradication program staffed by TB tracers, using many of the techniques perfected in its outbreak control efforts. By 1950, one out of every four houses surveyed had an active case of TB. This was particularly striking when compared to a rate of just 7.6 percent seven years earlier.[7] To understand this failure, I turn to two specific cases of health center efforts to treat TB to illustrate the health center's program and the trouble it had.

Treating TB through Social Medicine: Thembisa's Case of TB and Idliso as Political Ecology in Action

The PCHC's 1944 Annual Report offers an extended case study of TB in a "problem family." On a routine visit to the family's homestead, health assistants discovered a nonresident man, Sibonelo, coughing.[8] They took a sample of his sputum back to the health center, where they discovered that he had tuberculosis.

When the health assistants returned to the house, they learned that Sibonelo and the other residents of the homestead, including a family member who was an inyanga, understood that he was suffering from idliso. As a result, Sibonelo refused treatment, health center education efforts failed, and two months later, he died. The message is clear: belief in witchcraft led to death.

This account of Sibonelo's fatal TB includes many attributes of the household; it notes that the family's educational standard was extremely low, that food production was well below average, and that "little effort was made by the family to fall into line with the Health Unit's campaign for vegetable production."[9] Sidney Kark, who wrote the report, explained that though the health assistants had visited the home repeatedly, none of their suggested improvements had been implemented, and further that no one in the family visited the health center for examination or treatment for TB for well over a year after Sibonelo died. The frustration is palpable and the subtext is clear: not only did they believe in witchcraft, but this family was not a model of health center practice, nor were its members good research subjects.[10] Sibonelo's death was, at least in part, the family's fault.

The report jumps forward a year to when, in December of 1943, the family brought a young woman, Thembisa, from the household to the health center. Thembisa was desperately ill and wasting away. A sputum test confirmed that she was sick with tuberculosis. Because of the health center's familiarity with the homestead and Sibonelo's death, the doctors and health assistants quickly traced the source of infection back to this family and its homestead. With this information, the team put together a "programme of action" based on its understanding of TB, its knowledge of life in Pholela, and the specific household information it had gained through periodic (unwanted) visits to the homestead.

In 1943, the antibiotics that treat TB had not yet been used on humans. As a result, the health center treated the illness palliatively by addressing Thembisa's symptoms and boosting her immune system, and by working to stop the spread of infection for everyone else in her household. In this case, the PCHC first provided Thembisa's family with food and nutritional supplements in the form of prescriptions until they could earn enough money to buy their own. (Thembisa had fallen ill in December, at the start of the growing season, when household supplies of homegrown food were at their lowest.) These prescriptions of food, so central to the health center's nutrition program, helped to improve the baseline health of Thembisa and the rest of her family, thereby decreasing the chance that TB would spread in her body and in the family. Second, thanks to its knowledge of the sleeping arrangements, the team persuaded the family to bring many (though not all) of the people who slept in the same space as Thembisa to be tested for TB. And though her family did not want Thembisa to be hospitalized, they did agree to keep her isolated from healthy family members in a separate building at the homestead. Third, using its knowledge of Pholela's kinship network and the health status of other households, the team suggested that the various children who were not sick be sent to stay with relatives, thereby removing them from the source of infection. By knowing this family well and by knowing how TB passes (through the air, in confined spaces), the health center managed to slow the spread of disease in the family. Fourth, health center staff found employment on a local road crew for at least one of the young men of the family so that the family would have money to buy nutritious food. They also found financial aid for the family's children to attend school, in the belief that with an education, they would have a higher chance of supporting the rest of family in the future.[11] The free, nutritious school lunch was a welcome bonus.

As the health center's account reads, once it had treated this woman and her family for both the tuberculosis infection and the poverty, lack of nutritious food, and lack of education that underlay it, her health improved and the family was better able to care for itself. Moreover, once the family had experienced the benefits of the health center's programs, they began to incorporate health center teachings like planting a vegetable garden into their homestead and began to participate more regularly in health center activities. By implementing one program that treated the biological and social aspects of Thembisa's illness and her family's vulnerability, the health center enacted a perfect social medicine approach to TB. And in this case, it was successful; this "programme of action" improved the health of Thembisa and halted the spread of TB in her household.

From the perspective of the health center, this success was thanks to its comprehensive program, which addressed both biological and social aspects of illness, and thanks to the family's good choices and hard work. By being persistent and simply enacting the standard social medicine outreach and education program, this health center team had laid the groundwork for success once Thembisa fell ill. It was successful in this case in part because tuberculosis lent itself to an approach that combined an attention to the social determinants of illness and wellness (poverty and family relationships) and the biological or biomedical causes of illness (bacteria, malnutrition, and poor ventilation), which all came together in the household and the family.[12] It was a program that, in true social medicine fashion, enrolled humans and nonhumans to improve health. It was political ecology of health at work. It also failed most of the time.

Treating TB by Killing the Bacteria:
Khanyisile's Case of TB and Idliso

In 1949, the first antibiotics were used against TB in humans to great effect. They quickly made their way to Pholela, giving the health center another option in its treatment portfolio. Soon thereafter, around 1950, Khanyisile, a young married woman who was living in Pholela, arrived at the PCHC.[13] She was very sick. Health center doctors diagnosed her with tuberculosis and explained to her and her family that she had contracted the disease at home. (Khanyisile was newly married and therefore had recently moved to her husband's home.) Khanyisile disagreed with this diagnosis and refused treatment. Instead, she visited an inyanga for idliso. She followed the treatment regimen prescribed by the inyanga, but showed little improvement. Thinking that she had contracted a particularly strong case of idliso, Khanyisile left her new home and returned to her family's home (her premarriage home). Her family reasoned that because she was newly married, her new ancestors (her husband's ancestors) did not yet know her and thus could not sufficiently protect her from illness and could not help with her treatment. (She was still following hlonipha-related milk prohibitions.) They knew that her treatment would be more effective, and she would be better protected from illness in her premarriage home, where the ancestors recognized her. In addition, Khanyisile's family feared that the influence of abathakathi was too strong in her married home because that was likely where she had come into contact with the umuthi that had made her sick.

Soon after her return to her premarriage home, four people there became seriously ill and her father, a part-time inyanga, decided to visit the health center. There he met with John Cassel, the medical director of the PCHC. After listening to Dr. Cassel's TB diagnosis, Khanyisile's father offered a long lesson about idliso.[14] He explained to Dr. Cassel that idliso is an illness caused by an ill-wisher who hires an umthakathi to make an umuthi that will cause idliso. The umthakathi puts the umuthi in the food of the intended victim to make her sick; once the person ingests the food, she falls ill.[15] He explained that a person who is sick with idliso has a productive cough, a terrible pain in her chest, night sweats, a fever, and weight loss. These were the exact same symptoms Khanyisile exhibited. He finished by explaining that if a person who contracts idliso is not treated, she will die.

After completing this lesson, Khanyisle's father quizzed Dr. Cassel about his comprehension of idliso. Satisfied that the doctor understood the passage of illness, he (the inyanga) decided to follow health center advice and have his daughter hospitalized for TB. Elated, Dr. Cassel took the opportunity to explain to Khanyisile's father how tuberculosis spreads. In a sense, he was returning the educational favor. He explained that tuberculosis is caused by bacteria that pass from person to person through the air or through food. When a person like Khanyisile catches TB, the tuberculin bacilli (the bacteria) settle in her lungs and spread in her body. Dr. Cassel finished explaining that in its symptomatic phase, TB causes high fevers, chills, night sweats, a sore chest, coughing, and weight loss and could lead to death. These were the symptoms Khanyisile had, and the exact same symptoms as idliso. He took this to mean that Dr. Cassel was implying that Khanyisile must have gotten TB from someone she lived with and passed it on in the family. Upon hearing this, Khanyisile's father withdrew consent for hospitalization and left.

Where the health center saw rampant tuberculosis in Pholela, many of the people who were resisting treatment were suffering from idliso.[16] The most important difference between these two illnesses is their cause. Bacteria cause TB and witchcraft causes idliso. This contrast made for distinct experiences and treatments for the people who were sick; they made for different illnesses. In a place where ill people and their families determined what was making them sick (in this case, idliso or TB), what was causing their illness (witchcraft or bacteria), and which healer to visit (an isangoma and an inyanga or a doctor), recognizing all facets of an illness was particularly important. Taking all these factors into account, Khanyisile's father knew that his daughter was sick with idliso, even if she might also have had TB.[17] The treatments and prevention methods for idliso and TB are different, as they both relate directly to their cause. For tuberculosis, which is caused by a bacterium, the treatment in the 1950s was antibiotics (when available) and isolation to stop the spread of the disease. Once the immediate needs of the sick person and her family were addressed, the health center worked to improve the homestead, livelihood, nutrition, and health of the family in order to prevent future infections, just as it had in Thembisa's case. Through this approach, the health center addressed the health of people's bodies and the broader ecologies in which they lived in tandem.[18]

For idliso, caused by an umuthi ingested in food, treatment was a purgative so that an ill person would vomit the poison to free her body of the thing that was making her sick. This treatment required that she be at home with her family to ensure that she received good care and that her ancestors, who were buried in the yard, could help her heal and could protect her from further attacks of witchcraft. If a person did not get better from this treatment and she and her family still believed that she had idliso, she went to a different inyanga or back to the same inyanga for a stronger remedy. If these treatments did not work, the family would likely take it as a sign that their ill daughter either did not have idliso or was cured of idliso and also had something else. The family would then decide to move on to a different healer, such as a doctor, who would treat her for another illness like TB. This decision would be based on continued illness in spite of treatment. For Pholela's residents, the process for assessing and dealing with TB treatment was similar.[19]

Attending to the different worlds of health and healing from which TB and idliso emerge, Cassel's story offers important insight into the health center's failure with TB in Pholela. From the perspective of the health center in this new age of antibiotics, Khanyisile's only hope for treatment and recovery lay with the hospital, pharmaceuticals, and the health center's plan to remake the homestead. Even in the PCHC prevention program's relatively holistic approach, its treatment for TB had come to recognize *Mycobacterium tuberculosis*, a single agent, as the primary cause of infection. Of course, the health center knew that the bacterium was entangled with a broader social world (understood through political economy), but it also knew that its ability to intervene in the political-economic structures that made labor migration an inevitability and poverty a baseline was limited. As a result, the health center prescribed antibiotics and sought to separate sick people from healthy ones to prevent the bacteria from spreading. This treatment was designed both to rid the body of the bacteria and to halt the spread of disease in the community; both were directed at stopping the bacterial agent. In offering health education, while also removing the bacteria from the family and the community, the health center hoped that it could improve the health of the community long into the future.

For people who recognized idliso, however, the health center's approach seemed both odd and accusatory. In this story, when Dr. Cassel explained to Khanyisile's father how TB spread, he had effectively accused his daughter of witchcraft. After all, idliso is a witchcraft illness passed from one person to another with the help of an umthakathi; it is the product of intent, always entangled in the social world of family and community relationships. In explaining that Khanyisile had passed TB to other members of her household, Dr. Cassel had unknowingly accused her of spreading illness in her family.[20] Khanyisile's father knew that good daughters do not spread illness in their family and Khanyisile was a good daughter. For Dr. Cassel, witchcraft was not real and believing in witchcraft was a problem, proof of a population not yet educated.[21] Cassel saw this lack of education, not poverty, not racism, not a problem with the homestead environment, as the single biggest reason that TB rates continued to rise. By this logic, the persistence of idliso was a problem of culture, not a problem of the physical body or of political economy. The solution was therefore more scientific education so that Pholela's residents would understand their biological bodies and come to recognize that their cultural explanations were not real, at least not in any bodily material sense. This would then pave the way for antibiotics and other scientifically tested treatments; it would pave the way for success.

As in the case of malnutrition that Diana Wylie writes about, in blaming the failure of the TB campaign and his failure with Khanyisile's father on culture, Dr. Cassel was avoiding biological determinism. But his alternative smacked of cultural determinism. In this thinking, culture was the number one barrier to progress and health.[22] As Wylie argues, this thinking was a new form of paternalistic racism with a focus on the inferiority of African beliefs and choices instead of bodies.[23]

For Pholela's residents who felt the effects of witchcraft in their bodies, however, idliso was never simply about cultural beliefs; it was its own physical illness. In this understanding, the behavior of Khanyisile's father makes perfect sense. For her family, an umthakathi had clearly made her ill. Like bacteria, this was a single agent. Treatment therefore needed to directly address this cause of the illness. In this frame, the purgative prescribed by the inyanga, which caused Khanyisile to vomit out her illness and possibly even return it back to the person who sent it, served the same purpose as antibiotics did for TB: it addressed the single agent making Khanyisile sick.

Khanyisile's story did not end when her father withdrew his consent for treatment and left. Soon after leaving, Dr. Cassel tracked down Khanyisile's father and immediately backpedaled. The doctor quickly agreed that his understanding of TB was wrong, and further that the biomedical explanation for the spatial pathology of TB was incorrect.[24] In other words, Khanyisile could not be spreading TB in her family. This allowed Dr. Cassel to persuade Khanyisile's father to go through with the treatment for TB for his daughter, and she was hospitalized. This family might allow treatment, but they certainly were not abandoning the world of health and healing in which abathakathi make people sick.

Treating Tuberculosis, Rejecting Idliso

By 1955, a few years after Khanyisile's case of TB, six years after the introduction of antibiotics, and eleven years after the health center doctors wrote about their success with Thembisa, the TB program was still a failure.[25] In both Thembisa's and Khanyisile's cases, a family member became so sick that relatives saw no option but to bring her to the health center.[26] In each instance, the family had first visited a traditional healer and their homestead was far from ideal. Their family members were poor and malnourished and they had "backward practices and beliefs." In both accounts, the families included an inyanga (in Khanyisile's case, the head of the family was an inyanga), and both families actively accessed care from healers, not at the health center. It is clear from these write-ups that the health center located the difficulty with TB in the family and in problems with culture; these families had not embraced scientific social medicine, and the consequence was dire illness.

From the perspective of health center staff, achieving the promise of social medicine required scientific understanding and scientific practices. In both case studies, the health center had tried to intervene before the women became gravely ill. TB tracers, health assistants, and even doctors had visited the homesteads with biomedical lessons about TB, information on nutrition and other health issues, and approbations to improve the homestead. But the families had not followed the health center's suggestions and advice. The outcome was TB. Moreover, once an individual got sick, the families had been unwilling to isolate them. And as the infected person grew worse, tuberculosis spread. The implication was clear: the unwillingness to treat TB had consequences for the entire family and, by extension, the community. It undermined COPC.

In both accounts, it took the death of a household resident to motivate others to seek treatment at the health center. In each case, the health center's analysis was written after a diagnosis was made and a treatment plan created. These case studies presented the situation as though treating the ill woman for TB and only TB was the only option. In these accounts, it is clear that the health center staff hoped, even believed, that in experiencing successful treatment, these families would give up their backward beliefs, embrace the promise of social medicine, and abandon misguided ideas about witchcraft and ancestors—and more, that the health center's life-saving treatment would convince them that they no longer needed to visit izangoma (plural of inyanga) and izinyanga (plural of isangoma).

Make no mistake, these are conversion stories. As such, they reveal the health center's hope and belief that residents were trading the health and healing izangoma and izinyanga practiced for the health and healing the PCHC practiced.[27] As the health center saw it, conversion was the only sure way to better health. In some senses, they were right, at least in the stories chronicled here. In both of these examples, the families ultimately agreed to follow health center advice, and the women were successfully treated. The willingness of Pholela's residents to work with health assistants in their homesteads to build compost pits and gardens and to visit the health center for coughs and fevers did not, however, signal an abandonment of traditional medicine and the singular embrace of biomedicine. Nor did it indicate the adoption of social medicine's vision of health in full. Instead, it indicated a willingness on the part of Pholela's residents to enact two regimes of healing. Understanding illness through the stories of Pholela's residents reveals that health was multiple and so was healing.[28]

Recognizing the existence of both idliso and TB as different illnesses in Pholela roots this analysis in residents' experiences and understandings and acknowledges that witchcraft can make people sick, just as bacteria can. This follows the work of Stacey Langwick, who sees traditional medicine ontologically. In this case, it means understanding traditional medicine as a healing framework that addresses and (hopefully) improves physical illness. As these stories reveal, both tuberculosis and idliso had to be treated in order to ensure the health of the population. The failure of the health center to make provisions to treat idliso, to allow for the treatment of idliso, or to accommodate a mutual diagnosis surely played a role in the continued transmission of TB, just as residents' refusal to be treated for TB did. As these stories show, this short-coming in the PCHC's approach made residents less inclined to visit the health center with TB symptoms or to accept a diagnosis of TB. This approach led to the health center's failure.

Toward a New Understanding of Health: Thinking *through* Witchcraft

It should be clear by now that the PCHC's faith in and commitment to the bio-medical and social sciences contributed to its failure with tuberculosis. I could stop there, but doing so would risk reaffirming the idea that witchcraft represents the limit of biomedicine, rather than being another category of illness that affected and affects health in Pholela. An in-depth examination of idliso and how it works provides a vision of health centered on entanglements and an understanding of social life as more than human, which opens up possibilities for understanding physical illness more expansively. In thinking *through* witchcraft, as in examining witchcraft as a practice related to health, I bring together the work of various scholars who explore relational ontologies to understand health and healing as a world-making process.[29] Central to this work is a disruption of binaries like nature/culture, human/nonhuman, and mind/body, and a recognition that individual elements only exist in relation to one another. Put another way, these scholars posit that we are human because of our relationships with nonhumans (both inside and outside of us), that nature exists in its relationship to culture, and so on.[30] To understand Khanyisile's and Thembisa's cases of TB and idliso, I also draw on feminist science studies. This scholarship recognizes the ways in which relationships are not only central, but are irreducible. In other words, relationships are the basis of the worlds through which they are constructed, worlds that are "real," even as they are ever-changing, and even as they draw on and relate to one another. In using the term *real*, I follow the work of scholars from the ontological turn who "take seriously" the stories and explanations of their informants as well as work by indigenous and Africanist scholars to understand the worlds in which people like Pholela's residents live through their experiences and stories.[31] In the case of health and healing, this means understanding that beings like ancestors have real effects on the lives of residents. It means seeing these actors as shaping individuals and physical health through their relationships with other actors. In this rendering, it is the relationships that are constitutive of being that matter most.

Dissecting Idliso

Like all witchcraft illnesses, idliso is caused by an ill-wisher who hires an umthakathi to produce an umuthi to make a specific person sick.[32] There are any number of reasons to send an illness: jealousy, a desire for revenge, general dislike, and so on. To send idliso, one goes to an umthakathi because abathakathi hold specialized knowledge and have skills that others do not. Once commissioned, an umthakathi collects ingredients for an umuthi from the forest and from markets.[33] She then combines these ingredients while speaking over them, enlisting the help of her ancestors to make the umuthi potent. In the case of idliso, once the umuthi is produced, the umthakathi puts it into the food of the intended victim. The victim eats the food and contracts idliso. Once they do, they develop a sore chest, night sweats, fever, chills, and weight loss. The illness does not happen instantaneously and it lasts for quite a while. In other words, idliso is not just a reaction to the physical ingredients that make up the umuthi; it is not simply food poisoning.

In these examples, a person becomes sick as a result of the umthakathi and the umuthi. In the most direct sense, the umuthi makes a person sick. This idea of causation is like saying that a lack of nutrients makes people sick with malnutrition or that a bacterium makes people sick with tuberculosis. But witchcraft illnesses are clearly embedded in complex entanglements, which shape whether and how a person gets sick. Therefore, in order to understand idliso and other witchcraft illnesses, it is important to examine the specific social, material, and other components of imithi, and then examine how imithi make people sick.

An umuthi is made of a specific set of ingredients (usually plant and animal parts), it is prepared in a particular way, and it is combined in specific quantities.[34] The order of combining, the act of stirring, and the process of combination all matter in the production of imithi. This should sound at least somewhat familiar to those who take pharmaceuticals when ill, though in this case I am focusing on an umuthi that *causes* illness rather than one that cures. Pharmaceuticals are produced from specific chemical compounds developed by trained scientists according to a formulation that specifies not only the ingredients and their quantities, but also the way in which those ingredients are combined.[35] Similarly, the production of an umuthi involves ingredients, quantities, and a procedure for combining them. That said, even if someone who is not an umthakathi knew all of the ingredients in a particular umuthi and the correct procedure for production, they would not be able to produce the umuthi. This is unlike the case of pharmaceuticals where, at least in theory, anyone can be trained to produce them. By contrast, the umuthi requires an umthakathi, a person who sends witchcraft and who, as a result, holds specialized knowledge and skills often rooted in her family history. Unlike most other people in the community, an umthakathi holds the power to enlist the ancestors in her work and to inflict physical harm on individuals. Important for the potency they offer the umuthi, the ancestors are also important for what they reveal about the social world of witchcraft illness. In this world, ancestors trouble the divide between human and nonhuman as they transgress the boundary between the living and the dead, shaping the health and lives of their descendants.[36]

An umuthi's power comes from the fact that the umthakathi works with the help of her ancestors, the members of her family who have passed on, and from whom she has learned how to harm. A person's ancestors have significant power over illness and wellness. Abathakathi are therefore some of the most powerful people in a community. The same is true for izangoma, healers who work with the ancestors. For example, in the annual protection ritual in which families protect their homes and themselves against witchcraft illnesses, the isangoma enlists the help of her ancestors and the family's ancestors. Without the ancestors' help, the isangoma's efforts and her intelezi (the umuthi used in protection) would be ineffective. For an umthakathi, this is also true. The umthakathi talks with the ancestors while she is making the umuthi. The words she speaks, significant as a way to enlist the ancestors, are also important in and of themselves. In short, the umthakathi's incantations have power, material power, just as the ancestors have power in the everyday material reality of harming and healing, of health.

For idliso to spread, a number of specific people must be involved as well; it is a social illness in a narrow sense. Idliso is the product of intent. It will only appear if one person wants to make another person sick, which means that there must be some unrest in the family or in the community. For an umuthi to cause a person to have idliso, all of these conditions must be met. If there is no intended victim, if the ancestors do not help, if the specific ingredients are not combined in the right order, in the right quantities, at the right pace, if an umthakathi is not involved, and if she does not speak the right words, the person will not get idliso, even if she eats food with an umuthi mixed in. The person might get sick, but she will be sick with something else. Idliso is the entanglement of specific people, things, beings, practices, and relationships. If any element is missing, the umuthi will not be effective.

Health as Entanglements

This unpacking of all the components necessary for idliso highlights the importance of more-than-human entanglements for health. The concept of *entanglement* highlights inextricability; it offers a way to understand health (and illness) as relational from the start. To understand health as entanglement, one other concept is particularly helpful: practices. Illness comes into being through *practices* like harming and healing. In her work on atherosclerosis, Annemarie Mol argues that the notion of enactment, much like the idea of entanglement, allows for a focus on practice and process without pointing to a specific actor or group of actors.[37] Following this logic, illness and health come into being through practices even if not all of their constituent parts are recognizable, and even if it is not clear how they work. For example, I can recognize that an ill person has idliso, even if I do not know who placed the umuthi in her food, who sent it, or why and how exactly it makes her sick. Her illness and her good health are significant as they are enacted and experienced in symptoms, diagnosis, and treatment. As this example makes clear, the practices of illness and wellness are key to their existence. Returning to the case of Khanyisile, her idliso existed through the care and concern of her inyanga father, even if it is hard to trace how ancestors heal a person, and even if she also had tuberculosis. Practices and entanglements together are particularly valuable for understanding health in Pholela. Focusing on practices like the production of an umuthi, diagnosing an illness, and caring for a sick family member reveals that illness is the specific entanglement of matter and meaning.[38]

Following this logic, idliso, as an entanglement, is the product of the umuthi that harms, the physical experience of illness, social relations within and beyond Pholela, the isangoma's diagnosis, and another umuthi that heals. And all of these are the product of many, many more components. It is an entanglement born from the intra-actions of other entanglements. (Here again I follow Karen Barad, who uses the concept of intra-action to highlight the fact that beings are relational from the start.) This is where the idea of entanglements is particularly useful. Entanglements account for the intra-actions of all sorts of actors without a prescriptive account of *how* they interact. In other words, it allows for the possibility that witchcraft makes a person sick without necessarily knowing the direct causal pathways of illness. As such, entanglements offer a mode of thinking and a model of causality that not only accept but embrace uncertainty. Using this framework, idliso is the result of entanglements: a victim, her family, an umthakathi, an isangoma, neighbors, some plant and animal parts, an incantation, knowledge, ancestors, intentionality, and more are all entangled, causing idliso. Moreover, these different components come into being together, in relation to one another. This approach not only reduces the role and importance of individual components; it also questions the very existence of distinct components to begin with. If illnesses are entanglement, then idliso *is* the intra-actions of all of its components, which exist only in relation to each other. The exact temporal and spatial details of those entanglements— the exact, individual cause-and-effect chain—are not important, because idliso emerges from the entanglement as a whole. This entanglement cannot be mapped; it does not appear in an actor network or through a diagram because entanglements are co-constituted and emergent.

To understand health and illness in Pholela, and in sub-Saharan Africa more generally, where imithi are infused with things, knowledge, ancestral spirits, and other humans, nonhumans, and more-than-humans, entanglements are particularly valuable. In Africa, witchcraft illnesses make the divisions that have marked modern science untenable; they highlight the depth of entanglements between social life, biological life, and more.[39] Thinking through witchcraft leads to the realization that health is relationships, relationships which include more than people and things. In understanding and experiencing health as relationships, Pholela's residents offer a different reality, a different world, a separate ontology, rather than just a set of place-specific ideas. As such, the explanation of illness as entanglement is different from that common to medical anthropology, which focuses on the imbrication of culture and medicine (medical pluralism) or the role of political-economic forces in health (structural violence).[40] Through the concept of entanglement, the inextricability of physical health, political economy, and factors often relegated to culture is clear and ontological.[41]

Enacting Illness, Understanding Tuberculosis

By focusing on illnesses like TB as they are enacted through the practices of contracting, diagnosing, and treating illness, the lessons of idliso can be extended to illnesses categorized as biomedical. As I explained earlier, tuberculosis is caused by *Mycobacterium tuberculosis*, colloquially known as the tuberculin bacillus. This bacterium grows or multiplies in an oxygenated environment. Biomedical science teaches that the most common form of TB, pulmonary tuberculosis (TB in the lungs), passes through the air (which contains oxygen) when a person expels infectious droplets by coughing, sneezing, speaking, singing, or spitting. Another person in close proximity may then inhale the expelled droplets and the bacteria they contain, which settle in the lungs as the person breathes. TB can also be transmitted through shared food or drink, when one person consumes infected droplets left behind by another. The bacteria hold the potential for illness and the cough, sore chest, fever, night sweats, and weight loss that go along with it.[42] But for the bacterium (a nonhuman) to multiply and to spread, for it to make a person sick, it needs people. The bacteria increase inside lungs and other parts of humans and then perpetuate as they are passed through saliva. Without humans, this nonhuman would never spread. Whether or not a person becomes sick with TB depends on the number of infected droplets the person comes into contact with, the quality of the ventilation in the spaces she shares with others who are sick with TB, how often she is exposed and for how long, the virulence of the TB strain to which she has been exposed, and the strength of her immune system.[43] All of these factors depend on her access to resources, which shapes her ability to determine her housing, her diet, and possibly her access to medical care. In other words, as the PCHC recognized, infection is in part determined by racial capitalism.

For the health center, treatment for TB, at least in terms of social medicine, needed to reflect all facets of its cause, including the role of social life. Therefore, healing involved an attention to the political economy of the household. In the case of TB, South Africa's economy depended on migrant labor, which meant men traveled from Pholela to cities where they worked and lived in cramped quarters and contracted the disease, which they brought back and shared with their families and neighbors.[44] In addition, poverty had led to a poor diet and inadequate housing, which then led to a compromised immune system among residents and insufficient ventilation, which led to infection. In this model, A led to B led to C in separate, clear, and predictable steps. It was this model of causality that linked the social and the biological in the health center's world of health and healing and that led to a traditional political-ecology approach to treatment. If, however, TB is understood through the concept of entanglement, a different picture emerges. In this case, as with idliso, bacteria cause TB as they come into contact with people's bodies and the landscapes in which they live, both of which have been shaped by racial capitalism. The cause of illness is therefore the entanglements of saliva, poverty, bacteria, racism, immune system cells, and family ties. It is all of these elements at once as they relate to each other.

The treatment of the illness addresses these relationships, enlisting many different components: antibiotics, which themselves are the products of entanglements of chemical compounds combined in laboratories; corporations and governments that circulate and regulate them; doctors who prescribe them; family members who help monitor treatment; and ill people's immune systems, which help fight the bacteria. In addition, as in Thembisa's case of TB, the PCHC's treatment included prescriptions of nutritious food, new vegetable gardens, improved ventilation, isolation of the ill person, and employment and education. Treatment was all these things, even as it was not clear how they came together; it was the combination of social and physical attributes, a tacit acknowledgment of the entanglements of illness.

In this rendering of TB, the social and the biological are entangled—making a disease. Tracing the exact causal pathways that link employment to sore chests or education to antibiotics is not necessary for understanding that tuberculosis is the entanglement of intra-acting components. A focus on the entanglement of TB offers a different view of causality. It is a focus on relationships and inseparability. It is not about one distinct element interacting with the next interacting with the next; it is about mutuality and entanglement. Even though the causal chain cannot be traced, without these entanglements there would be no tuberculosis. In short, rather than view the various component parts separately as acting on one another, a focus on entanglements recognizes that they work in concert, often to unexpected ends.[45] Through an understanding of health as entanglement, effects emerge from relationships, and biology and social life are inseparable.

The Limits of Health Center Practice

Understanding illness and health as entanglements, and healing as practices, is important for understanding the PCHC's failures and the limits of social medicine. At the heart of the health center's failure with tuberculosis, in particular, was its inability to treat and even recognize idliso; it was the health center's inability to access a world of health and healing beyond its scientific focus, but one that nonetheless had material consequences for Pholela's residents. Part of the PCHC's frustration with its antituberculosis program stemmed from its remarkable success in other areas like maternal and child health, nutrition, and syphilis. Its success depended on its combined attention to what it understood to be the social and biological aspects of health, and a program attuned to addressing both. Residents' work, their understanding of nutrition and other diseases, and their incorporation of things like beetroot and new windows, were evidence that they and their bodies occupied a world of health and healing the health center could intervene in and improve.

But that was not the only world Pholela's residents and their bodies occupied. The failure of efforts to expand pit latrines and the failure of the health center's TB program are evidence of this. TB had something that malnutrition and syphilis did not: it had physical symptoms that matched those of a witchcraft illness. In Pholela, where the majority of illnesses were illnesses that just happened, this overlap was rare. In cases where there was not such a clear overlap, residents had no problem going to the health center. But when the symptoms were ambiguous, treatment became less clear-cut for residents, and one of the limits of the health center's social medicine program became clear; this is what happened when the anti-TB campaign met idliso. Understanding social medicine, and the antituberculosis campaign specifically, from the stories of people like Thembisa and Khanyisile in Pholela reveals that witchcraft illnesses represent an ontological reality that is different from that of biomedical illnesses, and further, that Pholela's residents live in ontological multiplicity. Understanding health through ontological multiplicity challenges scientific models of causality, positing that illness and health are the product of entanglements in which relationships are irreducible.[46]

The health center's fixation on the spatial pattern of the disease, its focus on illness at the homestead and community scales, and its understanding of Pholela, its people, homesteads, and communities, through a prism of biomedicine and political economy, all contributed to its inability to accept idliso. In these cases, the limitations of biomedicine's understanding of physical illness are easy to see in its singular focus on the bacteria. The limitations of the health center's social vision are just as easy to see. For the health center, racial capitalism was the social life that affected health by setting the broader context in which livelihoods and families were formed. By this thinking, key aspects of social life like poverty and labor migration meant that Pholela's residents were exposed to diseases like TB and that their bodies were not in shape to fight them off. Idliso, and witchcraft illnesses more generally, were rooted in different understandings of social life, in which an umthakathi, angry neighbors, ancestors, incantations, and plant and animal parts all inhabited the social landscape that made people sick. In addition, for these illnesses, the social life that made people sick was specific to the social world of the ill person; it was about their families, neighbors, ancestors, and homes. The very assumptions about social life and physical health embedded in social and biomedical sciences that had helped the health center succeed in making people healthier made it unsuccessful with tuberculosis.

The copresence of illnesses in Pholela and in residents' bodies reveals that ontological multiplicity connects the worlds of health and healing in Pholela through the lives and experiences of residents. As Annemarie Mol demonstrates, these worlds are often imbricated in one another; they represent ontological multiplicity. She writes that "the difficult aspect of ontological multiplicity [is] that while there is more reality than one, its different versions are variously entangled with one another, so that there are less than many."[47] Stacey Langwick brings this idea to the body, arguing that illness and bodies offer "moments of ontological coordination," where worlds of health and healing become visible.[48] Thembisa's and Khanyisile's stories of idliso and tuberculosis reveal that residents occupied and occupy multiple interconnected worlds.[49] They also reveal that the social life of health and healing for Pholela's residents was more expansive than it was for the social medicine developed in Pholela. The sciences that constituted the social medicine practiced in Pholela circumscribed what counted as social life, especially in terms of physical illness or the ontology of health. But the sore chests and coughing of people like Khanyisile and the concerns of residents who would not build pit latrines trouble those boundaries, laying bare the role of more-than-human social life in both health and illness.

Social Medicine in the Age of Global Health

In December 2015, I met the new medical director of the PCHC. A thin and well-built Zulu man in his early thirties, Dr. Makhanye was relatively new to Pholela. After greeting me, he told me that he had heard about my work and had learned a bit about the history of the PCHC, the COPC it developed, and its global impact. As we began chatting, I learned that Dr. Makhanye had gone to medical school in Cuba. Switching to Spanish, I asked if he had studied community medicine. "Sí, exactamente," he responded with pride. He said that the reason he had accepted the position at the PCHC was that he wanted to bring community medicine back to South Africa and thought that Pholela was a good place to start. But his enthusiasm had been tempered by the challenges of a health care system with little dedication to primary care (not to mention community care) and that was perpetually underfunded. He told me he was even thinking about taking a demotion and becoming a staff physician somewhere else because he wasn't sure the headaches were worth it.

As he saw it, the problem of South Africa's health care system and of medicine more generally was one of specialization. Doctors in South Africa are pushed into specializing in particular subfields of medicine such as cardiology or orthopedics, thanks to higher salaries and more prestige. Dr. Makhanye saw community medicine as the consummate generalist practice, in which the health of the person as a whole was understood and treated in relation to their community. It was about relationships both within the body and among people and households, not about individual body parts or diseases. According to him, this approach was the answer to the country's health care woes. He was talking about social medicine as the PCHC had practiced it.

Dr. Makhanye's critique was rooted in the PCHC of the twenty-teens. The health center was organized into separate wards, divided by health condition: an HIV/AIDS clinic, funded by international donors; a TB ward; a maternity ward; and a general care ward. The clinic's organization reflected the funding priorities of global health programs rather than the needs of the community. Under this organization, a pregnant woman who had diabetes and was sick with tuberculosis had to visit three different wards in order to receive the treatment she needed. This was certainly not medicine that attends to the person as a whole, let alone the person as a social being, in any sense of the term. Moreover, while the PCHC has a mobile unit that goes out into communities, it is made up entirely of mobile clinics that travel to a single point in a community where residents come to consult with a nurse and collect medications. There are also community health workers, funded by local NGOs, who visit their neighbors and offer health education with limited funding and training, but the days of a comprehensive community-based social medicine practice are long past.

Dr. Makhanye is not the only one concerned about a health care system that treats individual ailments, ignoring the body as a whole, and the social relationships that shape it. In 2008, I spent several months working with Dr. Smith in the PCHC's HIV/AIDS clinic, one of the government's first rural ART (antiretroviral therapy) clinics. He often commented on the trouble associated with having an HIV/AIDS clinic and a TB clinic separated from the rest of the health center. Dr. Smith, like Dr. Makhanye, saw a renewed focus on and investment in primary care as essential for reducing health disparities and improving the lives of South Africa's poorest people.

A number of prominent doctors worldwide, most notably Paul Farmer, have also called for a global health care system focused on primary care, in which each body is treated as a whole entity and people are recognized as parts of communities. And scholars of global health, including geographers, anthropologists, and historians have critiqued health care operations across the Global South for an approach that focuses on separate, often donor-driven and disease-specific operations at the expense of the whole person. Their critiques look at the roles of outside funding, weakened nation-states, and the wants and needs of powerful countries, which often end up being more important than those of the people and places they are purported to serve.[1] In some senses, these can be seen as critiques of the shift away from the social medicine practiced around the world during the third quarter of the twentieth century, a social medicine that was based in part on the pioneering work of the PCHC. They also echo Dr. Makhanye's observations, which were rooted in his experiences in Pholela and his training in Cuba.

Many of the health centers built on the Pholela model have been extremely effective, greatly improving the health of the communities they serve. But these are not institutions of global health. Their community focus and local specificity, not to mention their funding streams, differ from global health's efforts at universal solutions and evidence-based best practices, funded by governments, universities, and multilateral organizations mainly located in the Global North. Their effectiveness and their community base make them a good model for correcting some of the biggest problems with both global health programs and the medicine Dr. Makhanye described. And, as was the case in Pholela, the relationships between the health center and the community provide a foundation for health center work, as staff and residents work together to improve health. In addition, these health centers attend to the specifics of how racial capitalism both shapes the community as a whole and determines who gets sick and who gets better, and they develop treatment solutions focused on the whole person. This model would address many of the problems of global health that scholars have described. These are the lessons that the successes of the PCHC offer global health.

And yet a return to social medicine would still face the same limitations that it faced in Pholela in the time of the Karks. It would still be limited by the realities of racial capitalism and a vision focused on what it could make legible to governments and funders. And it would still understand health to be at the interface of the biology of the body and (human) social relationships, read through biomedical and nutritional science on the one hand and social science on the other. As the story I tell here demonstrates, understanding social medicine from Pholela offers a different perspective on health and healing, and a more expansive understanding of what constitutes social life. This perspective reveals that health is the product of relationships among humans, nonhumans, and harder-to-categorize beings like ancestors, and that causation is entangled. It also offers a vision of social life where relationships are irreducible. This is the key contribution of telling this story from Pholela, and from Africa more generally.

A return to the homestead offers a good starting point for imagining the different health care practices Pholela teaches us we need in the age of global health. One need only look at the water taps and beetroot alongside the graves of family members who have passed on and the intelezi planted in people's gardens to see that Pholela's residents continue to live in multiple worlds of health and healing. What these homesteads and the stories of people like Gogo Ngcobo and Gogo Sithole teach us is that health is something more than even the best social and medical science can explain. They teach us that the health of Pholela's residents and that of their neighbors is always rooted in multiple worlds at once, and further that there is not only more than one way to know health, but that there are multiple healths.

What does this mean for global health? The short answer is that this expansion of an understanding of social life may not offer much to a project of improving global health as a scientific practice. Instead, the lessons of social medicine understood from the homesteads, bodies, and lives of Pholela's residents and an ontological understanding of social life pose a fundamental challenge to the sciences that make up social medicine. Understanding social medicine from Pholela, therefore, leads to a different question. Rather than asking how we can make global health better, it pushes us to ask what conditions need to be met to ensure that everyone can be healthy.

This question leads to two important lessons: First, the solution to addressing the ongoing health challenges that result from witchcraft and ancestors lies neither in making biomedicine better nor in creating novel global health-related institutional arrangements. Embedded in institutions and their funding streams are assumptions about what constitutes results and what counts as success. These notions of success and measurement are organized according to scientific logics, logics that do not and cannot recognize all of the more-than-human entanglements that shape health and healing in Pholela. In other words, science underpins global health and undergirds clinical practice. For science, witchcraft does not exist. As a result, simply incorporating traditional healers into clinical care will do little to enact the vision of social medicine that Pholela teaches us we need. After all, it is hard to imagine that these illnesses and healers would even make it into the reports that global health programs write for their funders and for the public.

Second, examining health and healing through witchcraft highlights the lesson that health is relational and causality is entangled. And these lessons lead to different practices and different treatment regimens. Take the example of the epidemic of illness among the youth (people ages fifteen to thirty-five) in twenty-first-century South Africa, what Gogo Ngcobo referred to as "these diseases." While often understood as HIV/AIDS, the formulation "these diseases" indicates something more. In its plural articulation, it makes reference to the fact that in the first decade of the twenty-first century, the youth were sick and often dying from all sorts of diseases, including tuberculosis, shingles, pneumonia, meningitis, and more. In its translation as HIV, the common assumption is that these diseases prey on the bodies of people whose immune systems have been compromised by HIV/AIDS. But in Pholela, young people who died of chronic conditions like unchecked diabetes or a hypertensive episode or tuberculosis that they contracted even though they were HIV-negative also died of "these diseases." This is not just HIV.

"These diseases" also provides a way to articulate the troubles with and of youth in the postapartheid era. As such, it is a way to describe the failures of the state, the ongoing impact of racial capitalism, the disappointment of parents and neighbors, insufficient health care, and unmitigated illness. As Pholela's residents know well, the youth should not get sick and die. Their ill health is not only the result of a terrible virus and the microbes that prey on a compromised immune system; it is also the result of an inadequate health care system, unhealthy food, poorly ventilated spaces, a population weakened by poverty, and a state that should care about them but does not. For others still, it is the result of angry neighbors, the abathakathi they hire, the imithi they send, and the ancestors they call on.[2] This epidemic and the individual diseases that make it up challenge scientific causality. "These diseases" are devastating and are the result of relationships among people, microbes, the state and its newly enfranchised citizens, racial capitalism, processed food, angry neighbors, disappointed elders, uneducated youth, ancestors, healers, and more. In this articulation of the epidemic, an articulation *from* Pholela, the causal chains that science relies on are impossible to map. The epidemic is all of these things at once; causality is entangled, just as it is with idliso.

This understanding of what causes illness, of entangled causality, makes the scientific interventions that mark global health difficult. But rather than closing down possibilities, an understanding of entangled causality opens them up. In the language of science, this vision of causality leaves space for a better recognition of uncertainty in medicine. This uncertainty opens up possibilities for different models of causality and different modes of treatment. It offers a shift away from universal science to more place-specific programs, programs that attend to the details of the more-than-human entanglements that make up illness and wellness. Significantly, these programs would resist the urge to translate the ways in which the subjects of global health articulate their health and illness into biomedical terms; they would accept that physical illness can be attributed to people, ancestors, and witchcraft. The move away from translation poses a challenge to recent trends in medical education and global health that focus on training in cultural competency, which is the ability of medical and health practitioners to communicate biomedicine across cultural differences in order to more effectively treat people. After all, these are different illnesses, not different cultural interpretations.

Recognizing different articulations of illness as representing different ontological realities opens up new possibilities for treatment. This kind of practice would recognize the multiplicity of "these diseases" and focus on person-specific treatments to address the microbe making a person sick, that person's educational and employment opportunities, their relationships with their neighbors and ancestors, and whatever other forces might be contributing to their illness. It would foreground the relationships that make up the epidemic and the specificity of the ways those relationships make each individual sick. This practice is a radical departure from universal science and global health as it is currently constituted. An understanding of causality through entanglement decenters the germ and the job, both of which are so important to social medicine. In so doing, it allows for more expansive understandings of health and healing.

This approach is a different kind of political ecology, one that focuses on relationships and recognizes that social life is broader than political economy. This political ecology of health focuses on the specifics of a place and is not easily scaled up. Instead, it calls attention to the more-than-human, place-specific relationships that make people sick and that can make them better. It is a move away from a global health articulated through the metrics that funders use to assess program efficacy and targets for support. Yes, it requires an attention to the structural violence and medical pluralism that medical anthropology articulates, but it does something more. It requires a shift in thinking away from seeing non-biomedical healing practices as cultural artifacts to seeing them as a way to intervene in and improve the material world. As such, it is a call for a more capacious model for improving the lives and health of people like Pholela's residents. This is important. This broader, more comprehensive understanding might just make space for novel health programs that address the large gaps in morbidity and mortality that social medicine could never fully ameliorate in many places in the Global South. It might help produce more livable lives.

GLOSSARY

Throughout the book I have chosen to follow Zulu conventions for singular and plural. As a result, I have included both singular and plural to match the text.

amasi fermented or sour milk; a very popular, yogurt-like food.

gogo literally grandmother, though it refers to older women in general.

hlonipha literally respect; it also refers to that practice of following particular protocols like adhering to food taboos as a sign of respect.

idliso a witchcraft illness that has the same symptoms as tuberculosis.

intelezi a special umuthi used in protection rituals.

inyanga (plural: izinyanga) a category of local healers often referred to as herbalists. Izinyanga are generally male and heal by giving patients imithi that they prepare.

isangoma (plural: izangoma) a category of local healers often referred to as diviners. Izangoma are generally female and heal in consultation with the ancestors.

mkhulu literally grandfather, though it refers to older men in general.

umthakathi (plural: abathakathi) a person who practices and sends witchcraft.

umuthi (plural: imithi) a medicine or potion. An umuthi could be used to cure or treat an ill person, and it could also be sent by an umthakathi to make someone sick.

NOTES

Preface

1 "H. Jack Geiger, MD, M Sci Hug," n.d., http://physiciansforhumanrights.org/about
/people/board-emeriti/h-jack-geiger.html; "Commencement 2016: Biographies—
H. Jack Geiger," *TuftsNow*, 2016, https://now.tufts.edu/commencement2016
/biographies/geiger; Ted Henson, "Jack Geiger, MD, M.Sc. , Scd," *We Are Public
Health*, March 10, 2014, http://wearepublichealthproject.org/interview
/jack-geiger/.

2 He also founded Physicians for Social Responsibility, the Committee for Health
in South Africa, and the Medical Committee for Human Rights, among others.
And he was the Arthur C. Logan Professor Emeritus of Community Medicine at
the City University of New York Medical School when I interviewed him.

3 Martha J. Bailey and Andrew Goodman-Bacon, "The War on Poverty's Experi-
ment in Public Medicine: Community Health Centers and the Mortality of Older
Americans," NBER *Working Paper* no. 20653 (Boston: National Bureau of Economic
Research, 2014).

4 COPC became the central organizing principle of the Kupat Holim Health Insurance Institution—Israel's biggest health insurance scheme—in the 1960s, 1970s,
and 1980s. Since 1995, when the government mandated that all Israelis have
health insurance, it has become an integral part of all health insurance schemes.
J. D. Kark and J. H. Abramson, "Sidney Kark's Contributions to Epidemiology
and Community Medicine," *International Journal of Epidemiology* 32, no. 5 (2003):
882–84; Michal Shani et al., "International Primary Care Snapshots: Israel and
China," *British Journal of General Practice* 65, no. 634 (2015): 250–51.

5 For example, see H. Jack Geiger, "Community-Oriented Primary Care: A Path
to Community Development," *American Journal of Public Health* 92, no. 11 (2002):
1713–16; S. M. Tollman and W. M. Pick, "Roots, Shoots, but Too Little Fruit:
Assessing the Contribution of COPC in South Africa," *American Journal of Public
Health* 92, no. 11 (2002): 1725–28.

6 The university put this social medicine practice into effect along with the Ugan-
dan government, as the university established the Kasangati Health Center. As
was the case in Pholela, the staff used the health center's eighteen-square-mile
"Designated Area" as a "laboratory for community medicine," and as a place to
teach medical students how to practice community medicine. George Mondo
Kagonyera, "Research and Innovations in Makerere University and Prospects
for Strategic Partnerships between Makerere/Uganda and Unisa/South Africa"
(Kampala, Uganda: Makerere University, 2013).

7 Other students of the program have gone to places like Spain, Colombia, the UK, Uruguay, and beyond, to help establish community health centers bringing COPC to the poor the world over. And still more programs have developed at universities around the world, including a residency program in COPC at Canada's McGill University Medical School.

8 Along with other South Africans from the health center movement such as Harry Phillips, Eva Salber (at Duke), Cecil Slome (the third medical director of the PCHC), and Guy Steuart, many of whom had spent time in Pholela, John Cassel established UNC as one of the world leaders in social epidemiology and social medicine. Norman Scotch, an anthropologist and public health expert who completed a postdoctoral fellowship at the Institute for Family and Community Health in Durban working in part in Pholela, became dean of public health at Boston University, infusing that program with concerns about social life and social epidemiology. Zina Stein and Mervyn Susser, who had completed a short course in Pholela when they were medical students at the University of the Witwatersrand in Johannesburg, moved first to England, where they taught epidemiology at Manchester University, and then to Columbia University, where they established a leading program in social epidemiology.

9 In using the term *traditional healing*, I am following the lead of Stacey Langwick, who recognizes the downsides of the term and yet uses it because of its broad recognition and resonance. In a footnote to an article about the simultaneous use of traditional medicine and biomedicine, Langwick writes, "Referring to 'traditional' and 'modern' medicine is a historically fraught proposition. 'Traditional' medicine emerged in relation to the spread of biomedicine in eastern Africa. It has served as a catchall category indexing forms of healing, kinds of affliction, and types of experts that were not officially included in missionary or colonial health care. Traditional medicine, then, is all that is not modern medicine, or biomedicine. This initial collapsing of diverse healing practices into the category of traditional medicine undoubtedly did violence to forms of difference that were salient in colonial Tanganyika, but today references to traditional medicine are widespread. As the category has gained epistemic and bureaucratic weight over time, healers themselves have come to organize around their common commitment to and practice of traditional medicine. The contemporary life of the phrase traditional medicine does not make such references any less fraught, but it does make them important sites of inquiry." Stacey A. Langwick, "Articulate(d) Bodies: Traditional Medicine in a Tanzanian Hospital," *American Ethnologist* 35, no. 3 (2008): 437.

Introduction: Social Medicine from Pholela

1 In accordance with the Institutional Review Board, I have given all named research participants pseudonyms. I collected pseudonyms in consultation with the people who populate these pages, and in some instances research participants chose their own names. I did this in part because in Zulu, names reveal much about both the lineage of a person and where they are from. As such, Thokozile,

my research assistant and collaborator, and I thought it best to keep the names local, so to speak, so that readers familiar with this naming practice would be able to make sense of these names and their geography. In addition, I have given all communities pseudonyms to further protect research participants, and when attributing specific pieces of sensitive information or ideas to interviews I often omit the names of interviewees. Most interviews were conducted in Zulu and translated by the author with Thokozile Nguse. For a critical look at the practice of using pseudonyms, see Nancy Scheper-Hughes, "Ire in Ireland," *Ethnography* 1, no. 1 (2000): 117–40.

2 I've written elsewhere about "these diseases" in an article about TB and HIV. Abigail H. Neely, "Internal Ecologies and the Limits of Local Biologies: A Political Ecology of Tuberculosis in the Time of AIDS," *Annals of the Association of American Geographers* 105, no. 4 (2015): 791–805.

3 National Library of Medicine, "Community Health: A Model for the World," https://apps.nlm.nih.gov/againsttheodds/exhibit/community_health/model _world.cfm.

4 One of the most important and influential texts about racial capitalism is Cedric Robinson's *Black Marxism*. I go into this in more detail in chapter 3. Cedric J. Robinson, *Black Marxism: The Making of the Black Radical Tradition* (Chapel Hill: University of North Carolina Press, 2000).

5 Theodore M. Brown and Elizabeth Fee, "Rudolf Carl Virchow: Medical Scientist, Social Reformer, Role Model," *American Journal of Public Health* 96, no. 12 (2006): 2104–5.

6 Bertram Lord Dawson, "Interim Report on the Future Provision of Medical and Allied Services" (London: Ministry of Health, Consultative Council on Medical and Allied Services, 1920); N. T. A. Oswald, "A Social Health Service without Social Doctors," *Social History of Medicine* 4, no. 2 (1991): 295–315.

7 Henry E. Sigerist, *Socialized Medicine in the Soviet Union* (New York: W. W. Norton, 1937).

8 Thomas McKeown, "Determinants of Health," *Life* 60, no. 40 (1978): 3.

9 Sidney Kark and Emily Kark, *Promoting Community Health: From Pholela to Jerusalem* (Johannesburg: University of the Witwatersrand Press, 1999).

10 Victor W. Sidel, "The Barefoot Doctors of the People's Republic of China," *New England Journal of Medicine* 286, no. 24 (1972): 1292–1300.

11 For a critique of this focus, see Abigail H. Neely and Alex M. Nading, "Global Health from the Outside: The Promise of Place-Based Research," *Health and Place* 45(2017); China Scherz, "Stuck in the Clinic: Vernacular Healing and Medical Anthropology in Contemporary Sub-Saharan Africa," *Medical Anthropology Quarterly* 32, no. 4 (2018): 55–63.

12 The *American Journal of Public Health* dedicated most of an issue to detailing the story of COPC as rooted in Pholela. "Community Oriented Primary Care," *American Journal of Public Health* 92, no. 11 (2002).

13 Patrick Wolfe, *Settler Colonialism and the Transformation of Anthropology* (London: Cassell, 1999).

14 See figure P.1 in the preface.

15 Leonard Monteath Thompson, *A History of South Africa*, 3rd ed. (New Haven, CT: Yale University Press, 2001), 297.

16 Dorrit Posel, "How Do Households Work? Migration, the Household and Remittance Behaviour in South Africa," *Social Dynamics* 27, no. 1 (2001): 165–89; Cherryl Walker, *Women and Gender in Southern Africa to 1945* (Cape Town: David Philip, 1990).

17 Pholela had the second highest recorded level of labor migration in the country.

18 Steven Feierman offers an explanation of different illness categories, which seems to hold across various Bantu-speaking peoples. He notes that there are three categories of illness as well, though he refers to the category I have named illnesses that "just happen" as "illnesses from God." My choice of term follows from Harriet Ngubane's work on Zulu health and healing. I have chosen to call these illnesses that "just happen" because in my time in Pholela I never heard anyone refer to them as illnesses from God. While it is true that people would attribute many things to God, including illness in general, there was not a specific category as laid out in the framework here. Further, the idea of an illness that "just happens"—its lack of intentionality, and the element of surprise—seems most closely aligned with the spirit of this type of illness. Nonetheless, I owe a great intellectual debt to Steven Feierman and to other scholars like John Janzen for contributing to the framework I employ here for health and healing. Steven Feierman, "Struggles for Control: The Social Roots of Health and Healing in Modern Africa," *African Studies Review* 28, nos. 2–3 (1985): 73–147; Steven Feierman, "Explaining Uncertainty in the Medical World of Ghaambo," *Bulletin of the History of Medicine* 74 (2000): 317–44; Steven Feierman and John M. Janzen, eds., *The Social Basis of Health and Healing in Africa* (Berkeley: University of California Press, 1992); Harriet Ngubane, *Body and Mind in Zulu Medicine: An Ethnography of Health and Disease in Nyuswa-Zulu Thought and Practice* (London: Academic Press, 1977).

19 Health center doctors lumped both witchcraft and ancestor illnesses into a category they called "psychosocial" illnesses. This was their attempt to offer a scientific rationale to a category of illness they had no other way of explaining. That said, it is significant that they mentioned both ancestor and witchcraft illnesses, since their records offer documentary evidence that both were present in Pholela. 1944 PCHC Annual Report, National Archives Repository, Pretoria (SAB), Department of Health files (GES), vol. 1917, ref. 46/32; John Cassel, "A Comprehensive Health Program among South African Zulus," in *Health, Culture, and Community: Case Studies of Public Reactions to Health Programs*, ed. Benjamin D. Paul and Walter B. Miller (New York: Russell Sage Foundation, 1955); Kark and Kark, *Promoting Community Health*; Sidney L. Kark and Guy W. Steuart, *A Practice of Social Medicine: A South African Team's Experiences in Different African Communities* (Edinburgh: E. & S. Livingstone, 1962).

20 There is a burgeoning body of literature on political ecologies of health. For a good introduction, see Paul Jackson and Abigail H. Neely, "Triangulating Health toward a Practice of a Political Ecology of Health," *Progress in Human Geography* 39, no. 1 (2015): 47–64; Brian King, "Political Ecologies of Health," *Progress in Human*

Geography 34, no. 1 (2010): 38–55; Julie Guthman and B. Mansfield, "Nature, Difference and the Body," in *The Routledge Handbook of Political Ecology*, ed. Tom Perreault, Gavin Bridge, and James McCarthy, 558–70 (New York: Routledge, 2015); Brian King, "Political Ecologies of Disease and Health," in *The Routledge Handbook of Political Ecology*, ed. Tom Perreault, Gavin Bridge, and James McCarthy, 297–313 (New York: Routledge, 2015).

21 I explore the idea of entanglement and its usefulness for understanding health in chapter 4.

22 I take a lot of inspiration from Karen Barad's work. For example, see Karen Barad, "Posthumanist Performativity: Toward an Understanding of How Matter Comes to Matter," *Signs* 28, no. 3 (2003): 801–31; Karen Barad, *Meeting the Universe Halfway: Quantum Physics and the Entanglement of Matter and Meaning* (Durham, NC: Duke University Press, 2007).

23 The importance of relationships to the production of science is not new. I go into this in more detail in chapter 2. More specific to the question of medicine, medical anthropologists have long offered a critical look at biomedicine and how it is enacted, taught, and understood, recognizing it as socially constructed. For example, in her examination of the first medical school in Malawi, Claire Wendland demonstrates that far from the universal medical education one might expect from a school modeled on and accredited by institutions in the Global North, this medical school is deeply shaped by poverty, inequality, and traditional healing systems that students have experience with. The result is a Malawi-specific, or at least sub-Saharan African–specific biomedicine. Wendland, like many scholars of postcolonial medicine, teaches us that biomedicine and science more generally are culturally and geographically local. As we will see, and as was the case in Malawi, the social medicine developed by the PCHC was deeply shaped by the communities, homesteads, and people of Pholela. Sandra Harding, "Postcolonial and Feminist Philosophies of Science and Technology: Convergences and Dissonances," *Postcolonial Studies* 12, no. 4 (2009): 403; Claire L. Wendland, *A Heart for the Work: Journeys through an African Medical School* (Chicago: University of Chicago Press, 2010). For further examples, see Donna J. Haraway, *Simians, Cyborgs, and Women: The Reinvention of Nature* (New York: Routledge, 1991); Donna J. Haraway, *Primate Visions: Gender, Race, and Nature in the World of Modern Science* (New York: Psychology Press, 1989); Donna J. Haraway, *When Species Meet* (Minneapolis: University of Minnesota Press, 2008); Byron J. Good, *Medicine, Rationality and Experience: An Anthropological Perspective* (Cambridge, MA: Cambridge University Press, 1993). Also see Barad, *Meeting the Universe Halfway*, for an excellent analysis of the role of scientific apparatuses in the production of scientific knowledge and worlds.

24 My particular orientation to world making is rooted in debates about nature and society. I find these debates useful for two reasons: First, they led to or enabled a renewed interest in the material world, accounting for the relationships between humans and nonhumans within social theory and the social sciences. Building from this base, perhaps the single most important insight of this scholarship is that nature and society have always existed in relationship to one another,

and further that it was post-Enlightenment science that sought to (artificially) separate them. There are two major approaches to understanding nonhuman agency in science studies: actor-network theory and assemblages. Along with John Law, Michel Callon, and others, Bruno Latour developed ANT in order to understand the role of nonhumans like animals and bacteria in the production of science. In this theory, various actants (a term significant for its openness to nonhuman actors) are assembled in a network through which they are connected to each other. Their actions, intentional or not, affect the other members in the network in ways that are both predictable and unpredictable. Each actant is therefore shaped by the other actants both directly and indirectly, as causality in the network emerges relationally. Most importantly, ANT is processual, focusing on new actors and new ways of acting; it is fundamentally interested in agency and change, where agency is distributed among actants and change is cumulative. While the different actants matter, their relationships matter more, as all action, all agency, emerges through the network. An ANT approach could be valuable for understanding the health center's program to remake homesteads (the subject of chapter 3).

While this is useful for thinking relationally, a number of scholars have critiqued ANT for its flatness, which obfuscates power differences, for the fact that it doesn't sufficiently account for the researcher, and for the fact that it focuses on the collective, often at the expense of the individual. Drawing on the work of Deleuze and Guattari, a number of scholars offer the assemblage as an alternative way to think about worlds, agency, and causality relationally. In this thinking, all entities—assemblages and their component parts—are relational. These assemblages are heterogeneous and productive—they act in the world—and they are more than their parts. Put another way, assemblages are parts and wholes, which hold together through difference. As Anderson et al. write, "Assemblage privileges processes of formation and does not make a priori claims about the form of relational configurations or formations" (176). Assemblages are about the coming together—their relationships. Much as in an actor-network, assemblages are made up of distinct elements, all of which have the same ontological status at the start. Unlike ANT scholars, however, scholars who work through assemblages often trace power hierarchies, which emerge through the organization of and relationships in the assemblages. As a result, they see power differences as the result of relationships and as constitutive of relationships. The result is that questions of power are embedded in assemblages in a way that they are not in ANT. One aspect of assemblages that I find particularly useful for understanding health, healing, and social life is the focus on relationships and process without detailing causal pathways. (This is different from ANT, where relationships are mapped in a network.) In this way, an assemblage is valuable for understanding illness as always social and biological. Another valuable aspect of assemblage thinking is that a number of scholars see assemblages as an ethos of engagement, as a way to think about what might be possible rather than simply what is. This focus on engagement with the world opens up new ways to think about and understand worlds.

While valuable, for our purposes in understanding the worlds of health and healing that Pholela's residents occupied, assemblages also have their limitations. Most important is that though all action is relational and components change over time, assemblages retain their distinct, *individual* components. While the components at the end might not be the same as the components at the beginning, they retain some of their distinctiveness. While helpful, I find that this fidelity to individual elements does not fit perfectly with thinking through witchcraft, nor with thinking about research. Ben Anderson et al., "On Assemblages and Geography," *Dialogues in Human Geography* 2, no. 2 (2012): 171–89. Some key texts from these debates include Bruce Braun and Noel Castree, *Remaking Reality: Nature at the Millenium* (London: Routledge, 2005); William Cronon, *Uncommon Ground: Rethinking the Human Place in Nature* (New York: W. W. Norton, 1996); Carolyn Merchant, *The Death of Nature: Women, Ecology, and Scientific Revolution* (San Francisco: HarperSanFrancisco, 1981); Raymond Williams, "Ideas of Nature," in *Nature: Critical Concepts in the Social Sciences*, vol 1: *Thinking the Natural*, ed. David Inglis, John Bone, and Rhoda Wilkie, 47–62 (London: Routledge, 2005); Bruno Latour, *We Have Never Been Modern* (Cambridge, MA: Harvard University Press, 2012); Gilles Deleuze and Félix Guattari, *Anti-Oedipus* (London: A&C Black, 2004); Gilles Deleuze and Félix Guattari, *A Thousand Plateaus: Capitalism and Schizophrenia*, translated by B. Massumi (Minneapolis: University of Minnesota Press, 1987); Martin Müller, "Assemblages and Actor-Networks: Rethinking Socio-Material Power, Politics and Space," *Geography Compass* 9, no. 1 (2015): 27–41; Beth Greenhough, "Assembling an Island Laboratory," *Area* 43, no. 2 (2011): 134–38; Colin McFarlane and Ben Anderson, "Thinking with Assemblage," *Area* 43, no. 2 (2011): 162–64. Sarah Whatmore, *Hybrid Geographies: Natures, Cultures, Spaces* (London: SAGE, 2002). See also Sarah Whatmore, "Materialist Returns: Practising Cultural Geography in and for a More-Than-Human World," *cultural geographies* 13, no. 4 (2006): 600–609.

25 Using the example of epigenetics and toxins, Becky Mansfield and Julie Guthman reveal that the boundaries between bodies and their environments are never hard and fast; rather, they are imbricated in one another. Julie Guthman and Becky Mansfield, "The Implications of Environmental Epigenetics: A New Direction for Geographic Inquiry on Health, Space, and Nature-Society Relations," *Progress in Human Geography* 37, no. 4 (2013): 486–504; Guthman and Mansfield, "Nature, Difference, and the Body"; Becky Mansfield, "Race and the New Epigenetic Biopolitics of Environmental Health," *BioSocieties* 7, no. 4 (2012): 352–72; Becky Mansfield and Julie Guthman, "Epigenetic Life: Biological Plasticity, Abnormality, and New Configurations of Race and Reproduction," *cultural geographies* 22, no. 1 (2014): 3–20. See also Heidi Eileen Hausermann, "'I Could Not Be Idle Any Longer': Buruli Ulcer Treatment Assemblages in Rural Ghana," *Environment and Planning A* 47, no. 10 (2015): 2204–20; Becky Mansfield, "Environmental Health as Biosecurity: 'Seafood Choices,' Risk, and the Pregnant Woman as Threshold," *Annals of the Association of American Geographers* 102, no. 5 (2012): 969–76; Neely, "Internal Ecologies and the Limits of Local Biologies"; Becky Mansfield, "Health as a

Nature-Society Question," *Environment and Planning A* 40 (2008): 1015–19. For those unfamiliar with political ecology, the following provide a useful introduction: Raymond L. Bryant, *The International Handbook of Political Ecology* (Cheltenham, UK: Edward Elgar, 2015); Tom Perreault, Gavin Bridge, and James McCarthy, eds., *The Routledge Handbook of Political Ecology* (New York: Routledge, 2015); Paul Robbins, *Political Ecology: A Critical Introduction* (Malden, MA: Wiley-Blackwell, 2012); Dianne Rocheleau, Barbara Thomas-Slayter, and Esther Wangari, *Feminist Political Ecology: Global Issues and Local Experience* (New York: Routledge, 2013).

26 Robin D. G. Kelley, "What Did Cedric Robinson Mean by Racial Capitalism?," *Boston Review*, January 12, 2017; Robinson, *Black Marxism*.

27 Mark Hunter, "The Materiality of Everyday Sex: Thinking beyond 'Prostitution,'" *African Studies* 61, no. 1 (2002): 99–120; Mark Hunter, *Love in the Time of AIDS: Inequality, Gender, and Rights in South Africa* (Bloomington: Indiana University Press, 2010).

28 Stacy Leigh Pigg, "The Credible and the Credulous: The Question of 'Villagers' Beliefs' in Nepal," *Cultural Anthropology* 11, no. 2 (1996): 160–201. See also Patricia Henderson's work on AIDS and its impact on social and economic life: Patricia C. Henderson, "The Vertiginous Body and Social Metamorphosis in a Context of HIV/AIDS," *Anthropology Southern Africa* 27, nos. 1–2 (2004): 43–53; Patricia C. Henderson, *AIDS, Intimacy and Care in Rural Kwazulu-Natal: A Kinship of Bones* (Amsterdam: Amsterdam University Press, 2011).

29 Langwick argues that medical pluralism is insufficient for understanding different regimes of healing because it requires strict boundaries between them. She uses therapeutic objects and the practices through which they are used, take on meaning, and heal as a way to understand difference and overlap. My argument is slightly different, focusing on the ontology of witchcraft to rethink the meaning of health and illness (as opposed to healing). Stacey Ann Langwick, *Bodies, Politics, and African Healing: The Matter of Maladies in Tanzania* (Bloomington: Indiana University Press, 2011).

30 Feminist science studies and relational approaches more generally offer a way to understand the relationships between the biology and social life that make up health. In other words, they offer a nonbinary way of understanding health, offering a relational approach as an alternative to an understanding of health based on the separation of the biomedical and social sciences. For these scholars everything is relational—there are no distinct individual elements. As Donna Haraway writes, "Beings do not preexist their relatings." Donna J. Haraway, *The Companion Species Manifesto: Dogs, People, and Significant Otherness*, vol. 1 (Chicago: Prickly Paradigm, 2003), 6. See also Karen Barad, "Posthumanist Performativity"; Barad, *Meeting the Universe Halfway*; Haraway, *When Species Meet*; Whatmore, *Hybrid Geographies*; Whatmore, "Materialist Returns."

More specific to health, Margaret Lock and other anthropologists developed a particularly useful concept: local biologies. This concept asserts that the biology of health and illness is always entangled with the culture of a place; biology is local. For a further explanation, see P. Sean Brotherton and Vinh-Kim Nguyen,

"Revisiting Local Biology in the Era of Global Health," *Medical Anthropology* 32, no. 4 (2013): 287–90; Margaret Lock, *Encounters with Aging: Mythologies of Menopause in Japan and North America* (Berkeley: University of California Press, 1993); Margaret Lock, "The Tempering of Medical Anthropology: Troubling Natural Categories," *Medical Anthropology Quarterly* 15, no. 4 (2001): 487–92; Margaret Lock and Patricia Kaufert, "Menopause, Local Biologies, and Cultures of Aging," *American Journal of Human Biology* 13, no. 4 (2001): 494–504; Neely, "Internal Ecologies and the Limits of Local Biologies."

31 Stacey A. Langwick, "Articulate(d) Bodies: Traditional Medicine in a Tanzanian Hospital," *American Ethnologist* 35, no. 3 (2008): 428–39.

32 Just as I do, Langwick draws heavily from the work of Annemarie Mol. The idea of "ontological coordination" comes from her explanation of Mol's ethnography on arteriosclerosis in which the body multiple—the multiple bodies at work in diagnosis, treatment, and living with arteriosclerosis—offer "moments of ontological coordination," in Langwick's words. She draws on this idea developed around the body to think about the other objects of therapeutic practices and the landscapes from whence they come. Langwick, *Bodies, Politics, and African Healing*, 23. See also Annemarie Mol, *The Body Multiple: Ontology in Medical Practice* (Durham, NC: Duke University Press, 2002).

33 I offer a more complete argument about overlapping ontologies in an article about using objects to understand multiplicity. Abigail H. Neely, "Worlds in a Bottle: An Object-Centered Ethnography for Global Health," *Medicine Anthropology Theory* 6, no. 4 (2019): 127–41. In addition, see Marisol de la Cadena, "Indigenous Cosmopolitics in the Andes: Conceptual Reflections beyond 'Politics,'" *Cultural Anthropology* 25, no. 2 (2010): 334–70; Marisol de la Cadena, *Earth Beings: Ecologies of Practice across Andean Worlds* (Durham, NC: Duke University Press, 2015); Langwick, *Bodies, Politics, and African Healing*.

34 Scherz, "Stuck in the Clinic."

35 I take inspiration from Sandra Harding's work on feminist and postcolonial STS for this point. As Harding writes, "[F]eminism and postcolonialism both argue in effect that how we live together both enables and limits what we can know, and vice versa. Thus when new kinds of persons 'step on the stage of history' to rearticulate how they see themselves and the world, new kinds of sciences, philosophies of science, and epistemologies are both generated and also relied on by their listeners." Harding, "Postcolonial and Feminist Philosophies of Science and Technology," 403.

36 Vandana Shiva, *Biopiracy: The Plunder of Nature and Knowledge* (Berkeley, CA: North Atlantic, 2016), 8. See also Anne Pollock and Banu Subramaniam, "Resisting Power, Retooling Justice: Promises of Feminist Postcolonial Technosciences," *Science, Technology, and Human Values* 41, no. 6 (2016): 951–66; Angela Willey, "A World of Materialisms: Postcolonial Feminist Science Studies and the New Natural," *Science, Technology, and Human Values* 41, no. 6 (2016): 991–1014.

37 These community names are pseudonyms, chosen by people in the communities.

38 Thokozile and I have written about our experience conducting research and the

relationships that shape our practice elsewhere. Abigail H. Neely and Thokozile Nguse, "Relationships and Research Methods: Entanglements, Intra-Actions, and Diffraction," *The Routledge Handbook of Political Ecology*, ed. Tom Perrault, Gavin Bridge, and James McCarthy, 140–49 (London: Routledge, 2015).

39 Sarah Hunt, "Ontologies of Indigeneity: The Politics of Embodying a Concept," *cultural geographies* 21, no. 1 (2014): 27–32.

40 For examples, see A. T. Bryant, *A History of the Zulu and Neighbouring Tribes* (Cape Town: C. Struik, 1964); A. T. Bryant, *Zulu Medicine and Medicine-Men* (Cape Town: C. Struik, 1966); W. D. Hammond-Tooke, *Rituals and Medicines: Indigenous Healing in South Africa* (Johannesburg: Ad. Donker, 1989); W. D. Hammond-Tooke and Isaac Schapera, *The Bantu-Speaking Peoples of Southern Africa*, 2nd ed. (London: Routledge and Kegan Paul, 1974); Eileen Jensen Krige, *The Social System of the Zulus*, 3rd ed. (Pietermaritzburg: Shuter and Shooter, 1957); Monica Wilson, *Reaction to Conquest: Effects of Contact with Europeans on the Pondo of South Africa* (London: Oxford University Press, 1936).

41 For example, see Sidney L. Kark, *Epidemiology and Community Medicine* (New York: Appleton-Century-Crofts, 1974); Sidney L. Kark, *The Practice of Community-Oriented Primary Health Care* (New York: Appleton-Century-Crofts, 1981); Kark and Steuart, *A Practice of Social Medicine.*

42 Here I follow Karen Barad, who uses "matter" and "meaning" to articulate the relationships she is interested in in the production of science and worlds. Barad, *Meeting the Universe Halfway.*

43 Donna J. Haraway, *Modest_Witness@Second_Millennium.Femaleman©_Meets _Oncomouse™: Feminism and Technoscience* (New York: Routledge, 1997), 273.

44 Barad, "Posthumanist Performativity," 823.

45 Barad, "Posthumanist Performativity"; Barad, *Meeting the Universe Halfway*; "Interview with Karen Barad," in *New Materialism: Interviews and Cartographies*, ed. Rick Dolphijn and Iris van der Tuin, 48–70 (Ann Arbor, MI: Open Humanities Press).

46 This is, of course, old hat for people who conduct ethnographic research and feminist scholars more broadly. For example, see Sharlene Mollett, "Mapping Deception: The Politics of Mapping Miskito and Garifuna Space in Honduras," *Annals of the Association of American Geographers* 103, no. 5 (2013): 1227–41; Gillian Rose, "Situating Knowledges: Positionality, Reflexivities and Other Tactics," *Progress in Human Geography* 21, no. 3 (1997): 305–20; Farhana Sultana, "Reflexivity, Positionality and Participatory Ethics: Negotiating Fieldwork Dilemmas in International Research," ACME: *An International E-Journal for Critical Geographies* 6, no. 3 (2007): 374–85; Juanita Sundberg, "Masculinist Epistemologies and the Politics of Fieldwork in Latin Americanist Geography," *Professional Geographer* 55, no. 2 (2003): 180–90.

47 Thokozile and I wrote a piece about research as diffraction. Neely and Nguse, "Entanglements, Intra-Actions, and Diffraction."

1   For the most part, South Africa follows the British model of higher education, where medicine is an undergraduate degree.

2   PCHC 1945 Annual Report, National Archives Repository, Pretoria (SAB), Department of Health files (GES), vol. 1917, ref. 46/32, 58.

3   Unfortunately, I haven't been able to find the names of most of the health assistants. This says a lot about the people who wrote about the PCHC and who they imagined to be key players in the health center model.

4   Sidney Kark and Emily Kark, *Promoting Community Health: From Pholela to Jerusalem* (Johannesburg: University of the Witwatersrand Press, 1999), 8; H. W. Kanis, "Experiments in Social Medicine among Rural African Populations," in *Perspectives on the Health System: Economics of Health in South Africa*, ed. Gill Westcott and Francis Wilson (Johannesburg: Ravan, 1979). As I learned from talking with Mervyn Susser in 2008, the first health center in South Africa was in Alexandra Township, Johannesburg. Many medical students from the University of the Witwatersrand did some of their training hours there before Pholela opened its doors.

5   PCHC 1944 Annual Report , SAB, GES, vol. 1917, ref. 46/32; PCHC 1945 Annual Report, 46; John Cassel, "A Comprehensive Health Program among South African Zulus," in *Health, Culture, and Community: Case Studies of Public Reactions to Health Programs*, ed. Benjamin D. Paul and Walter B. Miller (New York: Russell Sage Foundation, 1955); Sidney L. Kark and John Cassel, "The Pholela Health Centre: A Progress Report. 1952," *American Journal of Public Health* 92, no. 11 (2002): 101–4; Mervyn Susser, "Pioneering Community-Oriented Primary Care," *Bulletin of the World Health Organization* 77, no. 5 (1999): 436–38; Cecil Slome, "Community Health in Rural Pholela," in *A Practice of Social Medicine: A South African Team's Experiences in Different African Communities*, ed. Sidney L. Kark and Guy W. Steuart (Edinburgh: E. & S. Livingstone, 1962).

6   James C. Scott, *Seeing Like a State: How Certain Schemes to Improve the Human Condition Have Failed* (New Haven, CT: Yale University Press, 1998).

7   The government began its efforts with research. The most notable and comprehensive reports from this era include the Native Economic Commission Report in 1932, which provided guidelines for development in the Reserves based on comprehensive research throughout the native areas of the country; the Native Affairs Commission Reports of 1937 and 1941, which offered more detailed information on native life; Sydney Kark and Edward Jali's Bantu Nutrition Survey; additional formal inquiries into aspects of health like tuberculosis and silicosis; and finally, the National Health Services Commission Report, which came out in 1944. To improve life for Africans, the government also established various new organizations and institutions, including the Ethnology Bureau, the Pholela Community Health Centre, and the Institute of Family and Community Health at the University of Natal's Medical School. Commission on Native Affairs, *Report of the Native Affairs Commission Appointed to Enquire into the Working of the Provisions of the Natives (Urban Areas) Act Relating to the Use and Supply of Kaffir Beer*

(Pretoria: Government Printing Office, 1942); Native Economic Commission, *Report of the Native Economic Commission 1930–1932* (Pretoria: Government Printer, 1932). Also see various reports from the Institute of Family and Community Health, available in the Rockefeller Archives Center (RAC), Rockefeller Foundation Collection (RFC), record group 1.2, series 487, subseries A, box 3.

8 Vincanne Adams writes about this postwar shift to a focus on health and economic development in the introduction to her edited volume, *Metrics*. Vincanne Adams, ed., *Metrics: What Counts in Global Health* (Durham, NC: Duke University Press, 2016). See also Helen Tilley, *Africa as a Living Laboratory: Empire, Development, and the Problem of Scientific Knowledge, 1870–1950* (Chicago: University of Chicago Press, 2011).

9 These new programs included the establishment of the Soil Conservation Service and the Soil Reclamation Program (what would come to be called Betterment), the roots of which dated back to 1934. William Beinart, *Twentieth-Century South Africa* (New York: Oxford University Press, 2001); Saul Dubow and Alan Jeeves, *South Africa's 1940s: Worlds of Possibilities* (Cape Town: Double Storey, 2005).

10 Much of the information in this section comes from accounts written by the Karks about their own histories, especially in their autobiographical *Promoting Community Health*. That said, the analysis in this section and its relationship to the rest of the chapter and the book are my own compilation, derived from the sources in the notes that follow. Kark and Kark, *Promoting Community Health*.

11 Of equal importance to their classroom teaching, a number of the faculty from the university's medical school held important posts in the South African government, and the Ministry of Health in particular. It was these men who would go on to champion Sidney, appointing him first to the Bantu Children's Nutrition Survey in 1939, next as medical director of the Pholela Community Health Centre in 1940, and then as head of the Institute for Family and Community Health at the University of Natal's new medical school in 1945. The faculty followed the careers of the Karks and visited them in Pholela and Durban, consistently supporting their efforts at community health. In addition, the medical school faculty would continue to be important for the Karks and their work even after they left Wits, serving as informal mentors as they developed COPC. In particular, the renowned physical anthropologist Raymond Dart, then dean of the medical school, took an active interest in the Karks and their scholarly and political work, championing them throughout their careers in South Africa.

12 Kark and Kark, *Promoting Community Health*, 7.

13 Some examples of the work of the faculty who had such a big influence on the Karks include Joseph Gillman and Theodore Gillman, *Perspectives in Human Malnutrition: A Contribution to the Biology of Disease from a Clinical and Pathological Study of Chronic Malnutrition and Pellagra in the African* (New York: Grune and Stratton, 1951); William M. Macmillan, *The South African Agrarian Problem and Its Historical Development* (Witwatersrand: Central News Agency, 1919); William M. Macmillan, *Africa beyond the Union* (Johannesburg: South African Institute of Race Relations, 1949); William M. Macmillan, *Africa Emergent: A Survey of Social, Political, and Eco-*

nomic Trends in British Africa (Harmondsworth, UK: Penguin Books, 1949); William M. Macmillan, *The Road to Self-Rule: A Study in Colonial Evolution* (London: Faber and Faber, 1959); William M. Macmillan, *The South African Agrarian Problem and Its Historical Development* (Pretoria: State Library, 1974); William M. Macmillan and John Philip, *Bantu, Boer, and Briton: The Making of the South African Native Problem*, rev. ed. (Oxford: Clarendon Press, 1963); J. D. Rheinallt Jones, Clement Martyn Doke, and D. F. Bleek, *Bushmen of the Southern Kalahari* (Johannesburg: University of the Witwatersrand Press, 1937); J. D. Rheinallt Jones and Ambrose Lynn Saffery, *Social and Economic Conditions of Native Life in the Union of South Africa: Findings of the Native Economic Commission, 1930–1932* (Johannesburg: University of the Witwatersrand Press, 1935); J. D. Rheinallt Jones and Reinhold Friedrich Alfred Hoernlé, *The Union's Burden of Poverty* (Johannesburg: South African Institute of Race Relations, 1942); J. D. Rheinallt Jones and Winifred Hoernlé, *At the Crossroad* (Johannesburg: South African Institute of Race Relations, 1953).

14   The South African Institute of Race Relations, established in 1929, was the first national multiracial organization to conduct socioeconomic research about race relations in South Africa. To this day it is known for its liberal politics and rigorous research.

15   Sidney was involved in the National Union of South African Students (NUSAS), an inclusive, nonracist, and nonsexist student organization with chapters at a number of universities. By the 1960s, NUSAS would become one of the most important anti-apartheid organizations in the country. That said, by the height of the anti-apartheid struggle, black students, most famously Steve Biko, criticized the organization for its white leadership and focus on white concerns. As a result, he and others created a nonwhite alternative student organization called the South African Student Organization (SASO). Coincidentally, Biko was studying at the country's first black medical school—the University of Natal's medical school—which had been started in part by the Karks. See "Freedom Day Struggle Heroes: Steve Biko and Donald James Woods," *YouTube*, April 28, 2015, https://www.youtube.com/watch?v=cPHTxiDcW8o.

Sidney eventually became leader of the NUSAS Labour Party and vice president of the entire organization. In addition, both he and Emily were involved in the Student Medical Council, of which Sidney was council chairman. And in the mid-1930s, they had founded the Society of Medical Conditions among the Bantu, which was the first organization to focus explicitly on the health of South Africa's majority African population. Like all medical schools in South Africa, the medical school at the University of the Witwatersrand was for white students only; the Karks' decision to create a medical society with a specific and explicit interest in the life and health of the African population was a radical move. Even in their student days, medicine and politics were necessarily intertwined for the Karks. There seems to be some disagreement on when the Karks founded the society, with Susser putting the date at 1936–37 and James Trostle putting it at 1934. Susser, "Pioneering Community-Oriented Primary Care," vi; James A. Trostle, *Epidemiology and Culture* (New York: Cambridge University Press, 2005), 27.

16 Diana Wylie, *Starving on a Full Stomach: Hunger and the Triumph of Cultural Racism in Modern South Africa* (Charlottesville: University Press of Virginia, 2001), 149.

17 Delimiting and bounding a study is a key component of all research. In science studies, scholars refer to things like community for the PCHC or a disease like AIDS for many global health projects as a boundary object. The boundary object becomes the center of study because it allows a number of different scientific communities to share information. This was certainly the case in Pholela, where a focus on community enabled the coming together of biomedicine and social science. Thanks to Laura Ogden for pointing out that the community was a boundary object. Joan H. Fujimura, "Crafting Science: Standardized Packages, Boundary Objects, and 'Translation,'" *Science as Practice and Culture* 168, no. 1992 (1992): 168–69; Susan Leigh Star and James R. Griesemer, "Institutional Ecology, 'Translations' and Boundary Objects: Amateurs and Professionals in Berkeley's Museum of Vertebrate Zoology, 1907–39," *Social Studies of Science* 19, no. 3 (1989): 387–420.

18 In place of the local name for the River View Area, I use the pseudonym Enkangala. Curiously, all other communities to be incorporated into the Designated Area kept their local names. PCHC 1945 Annual Report.

19 Arun Agrawal and Clark C. Gibson, "Enchantment and Disenchantment: The Role of Community in Natural Resource Conservation," *World Development* 27, no. 4 (1999): 629–49.

20 A number of scholars have written about the importance of meaning making through maps and other spatial practices. Scholars argue that maps and map-making help to make the world; they do not simply represent it. This perspective is particularly important for understanding Pholela, where the maps the health center produced were fundamental to making their work—and Pholela—legible to the government and later to funders like the Rockefeller Foundation. Derek Gregory, *Geographical Imaginations* (Cambridge, MA: Blackwell, 1994); J. Brian Harley, "Deconstructing the Map," *Cartographica: The International Journal for Geographic Information and Geovisualization* 26, no. 2 (1989): 1–20; J. Brian Harley, *The New Nature of Maps: Essays in the History of Cartography* (Baltimore: Johns Hopkins University Press, 2002); J. Brian Harley, "Maps, Knowledge, and Power," in *Geographic Thought: A Praxis Perspective*, ed. George L. Henderson and Marvin Waterstone, 129–48 (Abingdon, UK: Routledge, 2009); Peter Jackson, *Maps of Meaning* (London: Routledge, 2012); Henri Lefebvre, *The Production of Space*, translated by Donald Nicholson-Smith (Oxford: Blackwell, 1991).

21 Jane I. Guyer, "Household and Community in African Studies," *African Studies Review* 24, nos. 2–3 (1981): 87.

22 Agrawal and Gibson, "Enchantment and Disenchantment." Scholars also note that communities are often the site of contestation and cooperation among the people who live in them and between residents and the government. Allen Isaacman, "Peasants and Rural Social Protest in Africa," *African Studies Review* 33, no. 2 (1990): 1–120.

23 More recently, Crystal Biruk and Dana Prince have examined the use of the term

community by academics and practitioners in global public health programs. For global health experts, community is not about social relations and power struggles in a particular place, but is a term used to connote something more local and different from the universal, objective, expert work of global health. This was not the case in Pholela. For the PCHC, the community was constitutive of the social medicine—*community*-oriented primary care—developed in Pholela. Crystal Biruk and Dana Prince, "'Subjects, Participants, Collaborators,'" *International Feminist Journal of Politics* 10, no. 2 (2008): 236–46.

24 As Kark later wrote, "Defining the household of this area and allocating an address to each was an early task. There was much discussion with the people concerned, not only as to the purposes of introducing a health center address system, but also as to the use and functions of area maps, and what they considered to be a homestead. Homesteads often consisted of a number of nuclear family units. Each of these units lived in separate groups of huts within a homestead of an extended or joint family. Using field compasses, we located each homestead on the map, gave it an address, and recorded the census of each family within it." Sidney L. Kark, *The Practice of Community-Oriented Primary Health Care* (New York: Appleton-Century-Crofts, 1981), 199.

25 Guyer, "Household and Community in African Studies."

26 John Lambert writes about the household in South Africa specifically. John Lambert, *Betrayed Trust: Africans and the State in Colonial Natal* (Scottsville: University of Kwazulu Natal Press, 1995).

27 Guyer, "Household and Community in African Studies," 103.

28 SAB, Department of National Welfare (VWN) vol. 1002, ref. SW430/15, G. W. Gale, "The Training of Health Assistants as Health Educators," 194; PCHC 1945 Annual Report, 45; Sidney L. Kark, *Epidemiology and Community Medicine* (New York: Appleton-Century-Crofts, 1974), 273; PCHC 1944 Annual Report, 26.

29 The Designated Area expanded each year, geographically from the center, to include more homes. It expanded from 887 persons (139 homes) in 1942 to 5,000 in 1945 to 8,500 (1,045 homes) in 1951 and to 10,500 (1,300 homes) in 1957. Kark and Kark, *Promoting Community Health*, 42.

30 In some senses, I used a similar technique in my own research, conducting intensive fieldwork in two communities in the PCHC's Designated Area and one some forty-five kilometers away. This, I believe, allowed me to see what changes were the result of the PCHC and what were the result of other factors in Pholela or outside. In this social science research design, my logic was much like that of the health center. I wanted a "control" I could use for comparative purposes. Of course, I quickly discovered that the richness and meanings of the different places meant that the idea of a controlled study made little sense. Nonetheless, this was my original idea. In the next chapter, I explore my own research process more deeply as well as the limits of this thinking.

31 For example, see Peter J. Taylor, *Unruly Complexity: Ecology, Interpretation, Engagement* (Chicago: University of Chicago Press, 2010).

32 Jane I. Guyer et al., "Introduction: Number as Inventive Frontier," *Anthropological*

Theory 10, nos. 1–2 (2010): 36–61; Martha Lampland and Susan Leigh Star, *Standards and Their Stories: How Quantifying, Classifying, and Formalizing Practices Shape Everyday Life* (Ithaca, NY: Cornell University Press, 2009); Bruno Latour, *We Have Never Been Modern* (Cambridge, MA: Harvard University Press, 2012).

33   Scott, *Seeing Like a State*. This notion of data is also important in Michel Foucault's work, especially in his notion of "biopower." For example, see Michel Foucault, *The Birth of the Clinic: An Archaeology of Medical Perception* (New York: Pantheon, 1973); Michel Foucault, *The History of Sexuality: An Introduction*, vol. I, translated by Robert Hurley (New York: Vintage, 1990).

34   The minister of health referred to Pholela as a "laboratory for health centre work." SAB, GES vol. 2704, ref. 2/62, "Pholela Centre Provides 'Pilot Plan' for Native Health Schemes" (newspaper article), March 10, 1945.

35   *Metrics* is an important volume that investigates the role of metrics and the research that underpins them from a number of angles. While focused on global health, as opposed to earlier forms of health development like the PCHC, it offers much to think about in terms of the role of the production of social science knowledge in health care today. Adams, *Metrics*. Also see Johanna Tayloe Crane, *Scrambling for Africa: AIDS, Expertise, and the Rise of American Global Health Science* (Ithaca, NY: Cornell University Press, 2013); Crystal Biruk, *Cooking Data: Culture and Politics in an African Research World* (Durham, NC: Duke University Press, 2018).

36   Crystal Biruk, "Seeing Like a Research Project: Producing 'High-Quality Data' in AIDS Research in Malawi," *Medical Anthropology* 31, no. 4 (2012): 347–66, 352.

37   A number of other scholars have written about the process of turning complex reality into simplified numbers. For example, see Martha Lampland, "False Numbers as Formalizing Practices," *Social Studies of Science* 40, no. 3 (2010): 377–404; Lampland and Star, *Standards and Their Stories*.

38   Nolwazi Mkhwanazi, "Medical Anthropology in Africa: The Trouble with a Single Story," *Medical Anthropology* 35, no. 2 (2016): 193–202.

39   João Biehl and Adriana Petryna, *When People Come First: Critical Studies in Global Health* (Princeton, NJ: Princeton University Press, 2013); Adams, *Metrics*; Biruk, *Cooking Data*.

40   Guyer et al., "Introduction: Number as Inventive Frontier."

41   In addition to reading PCHC publications, I learned about the process of attending the health center through conversations with older people in the area.

42   When I arrived in Pholela in 2008, the original clinic had just been demolished. To my knowledge the last remaining files were inside that clinic. One of Pholela's residents showed me what she called the family file, but it was from after 1960 and it was quite different from what the Karks describe in their writings about the health center (it contained only a list of people and their diagnoses by the health center, no information on the homestead or broader familial relationships). As a result, I do not think it is representative of the family files that the Karks and their team used.

This particular annex from the 1944 Annual Report offers rich material for understanding how the health center viewed Pholela's families. That said, one must be careful to attend to what of the writing represented the actual feelings and opinions of the PCHC staff and what represented the staff writing for an audience that would expect them to take a particular position on topics like infidelity. Given discussions with public health and medical researchers who worked at the PCHC, I think it is likely that at least some of what the health center wrote about its misgivings about adultery were the result of its anticipated audience, rather than the opinion of any of its staff. 1944 Annual Report, 48–49.

43 1944 Annual Report, 49.

44 Byron J. Good, *Medicine, Rationality and Experience: An Anthropological Perspective* (Cambridge: Cambridge University Press, 1993).

45 Neil Brenner, "Urban Governance and the Production of New State Spaces in Western Europe, 1960–2000," *Review of International Political Economy* 11, no. 3 (2004): 447–88; Richard Howitt, "Scale as Relation: Musical Metaphors of Geographical Scale," *Area* 30, no. 1 (1998): 49–58; Sallie A. Marston, "The Social Construction of Scale," *Progress in Human Geography* 24, no. 2 (2000): 219–42; Robert B. McMaster and Eric Sheppard, "Introduction: Scale and Geographic Inquiry," in *Scale and Geographic Inquiry: Nature, Society, and Method*, ed. Robert B. McMaster and Eric Sheppard, 1–22 (Malden, MA: Blackwell, 2004); Erik Swyngedouw, "Neither Global nor Local: 'Glocalization' and the Politics of Scale," in *Space of Globalization: Reasserting the Power of the Local*, ed. Erik Swyngedouw, 115–36 (New York: Guilford/Longman, 1997).

46 Marston, "The Social Construction of Scale," 220.

47 In reflecting on health center practice, Kark wrote, "The whole process of the health center's development was one which reflected an increasing understanding of the individual in terms of his family situation, of the family in its life situation within the local community and finally the way of life of the community itself in relation to the social structure of South Africa." Sidney L. Kark, "Health Centre Service," in *Social Medicine*, ed. F. H. Cluver (Johannesburg: Central News Agency, 1951), 677.

48 1944 Annual Report, 49.

49 One could argue that this was an early recognition of the condition later articulated as "structural violence." Physician, anthropologist, and global health activist Paul Farmer is the scholar most clearly associated with the idea when it comes to health. I offer two articles (one with commentaries) on the topic, though any of Farmer's work helps to illustrate the idea. I take up structural violence in chapter 3. Paul Farmer, "On Suffering and Structural Violence: A View from Below," *Daedalus* 125, no. 1 (1996): 261–83; Paul Farmer et al., "An Anthropology of Structural Violence 1," *Current Anthropology* 45, no. 3 (2004): 305–25.

50 This was also an early version of the verbal or social autopsy used by epidemiologists today. Special thanks to one of the reviewers for pointing this out.

51 1944 Annual Report, annex A.

52 Vinay Kumar and Stanley L. Robbins, *Robbins Basic Pathology*, 8th ed. (Philadelphia: Saunders/Elsevier, 2007).

53 The health center's use of maps and its practice of containment and treatment was

the best public health practice of the time. As Yach and Tollman point out, spatial bounding and designation were central to public health thinking in South Africa in the 1940s and 1950s. D. Yach and S. M. Tollman, "Public Health Initiatives in South Africa in the 1940s and 1950s: Lessons for a Post-Apartheid Era," *American Journal of Public Health* 83, no. 7 (1993): 1043–50. See also Eustace Henry Cluver, *Public Health in South Africa*, 5th ed. (Johannesburg: Central News Agency, 1948).

54 Marston, "The Social Construction of Scale"; Sallie A. Marston, John Paul Jones III, and Keith Woodward, "Human Geography without Scale," *Transactions of the Institute of British Geographers* 30, no. 4 (2005): 416–32.

55 1951 Annual Report, SAB, GES, vol. 1917, ref. 46/32, annexure A.

56 1945 Annual Report, 59.

57 The PCHC's annual reports speak of the work they did to assist in other areas of the province, and the National Health Services Commission report modeled much of its recommendations on Pholela. Monthly and annual reports can be found in SAB, GES vol. 1917, ref. 46/32; GES vol. 2704, ref. 1/62; GES vol. 2704, ref. 2/62. Also see Henry Gluckman, *Report of the National Health Services Commission on the Provision of an Organized National Health Service for All Sections of the People of the Union of South Africa, 1942–1944* (Pretoria: Government Printer, 1944).

Chapter 2: Relationships and Social Medicine

1 This is a key lesson from Crystal Biruk's work on gathering data and conducting research around HIV/AIDS—research subjects (in this case, Pholela's residents) shape research and reality through their frequent interaction with researchers (in this case, PCHC staff). Crystal Biruk, *Cooking Data: Culture and Politics in an African Research World* (Durham, NC: Duke University Press, 2018).

2 Donald S. Moore, "Subaltern Struggles and the Politics of Place: Remapping Resistance in Zimbabwe's Eastern Highlands," *Cultural Anthropology* 13, no. 3 (1998): 344–81.

3 This was particularly striking when later compared to other research participants who appeared quite concerned that they get the answers right or that they tell us what we wanted to hear. In addition, this is a personality trait that Gogo Sithole is well known for—many of her friends and family members comment on it.

4 Many scholars have written about this. For example, see Deirdre McKay, "Negotiating Positionings: Exchanging Life Stories in Research Interviews," in *Feminist Geography in Practice: Research and Methods*, ed. Pamela Moss (Oxford: Blackwell, 2002); Joe Soss, "Talking Our Way to Meaningful Explanations: A Practice-Centered View of Interviewing for Interpretive Research," in *Interpretation and Method: Empirical Methods and the Interpretive Trend*, ed. Dvorra Yarrow and Peregrine Schwartz-Shea, 193–214 (New York: Routledge, 2015).

5 Caitlin Cahill, Farhana Sultana, and Rachel Pain, "Participatory Ethics: Politics, Practices, Institutions," *ACME: An International E-Journal for Critical Geographies* 6, no. 3 (2007): 304–18; Mike Crang, "Qualitative Methods: Touchy, Feely, Look-See?," *Progress in Human Geography* 27, no. 4 (2003): 494–504; Audrey Kobayashi, "Coloring the Field: Gender, 'Race,' and the Politics of Fieldwork," *Professional*

Geographer 46, no. 1 (1994): 73–80; Heidi J. Nast, "Women in the Field: Critical Feminist Methodologies and Theoretical Perspectives," *Professional Geographer* 46, no. 1 (1994): 54–66; Lynn A. Staeheli and Victoria A. Lawson, "Feminism, Praxis, and Human Geography," *Geographical Analysis* 27, no. 4 (1995): 321–38; Juanita Sundberg, "Masculinist Epistemologies and the Politics of Fieldwork in Latin Americanist Geography," *Professional Geographer* 55, no. 2 (2003): 180–90.

6 This (naive) thought on my part was the result of my efforts at reflexivity. Reflexivity is a practice that feminist scholars offer of reflecting on one's positionality as a way to think through how the researcher shapes the research encounter. Crang, "Qualitative Methods"; Kobayashi, "Coloring the Field"; Linda McDowell, "Doing Gender: Feminism, Feminists and Research Methods in Human Geography," *Transactions of the Institute of British Geographers* 17, no. 4 (1992): 399–416; Meghan Cope, "Feminist Epistemology in Geography," in *Feminist Geography in Practice: Research and Methods*, ed. Pamela Moss (Oxford: Blackwell, 2002); Cahill, Sultana, and Pain, "Participatory Ethics."

7 For more on the messy reality of power, relationships, and research, in my work in Pholela in particular, see Abigail H. Neely and Thokozile Nguse, "Relationships and Research Methods: Entanglements, Intra-Actions, and Diffraction," in *The Routledge Handbook of Political Ecology*, ed. Tom Perrault, Gavin Bridge, and James McCarthy, 140–49 (London: Routledge, 2015).

8 A number of scholars have written about the importance of developing standards. In the introduction to *Standards and Stories*, Susan Leigh Star and Martha Lampland write that "[s]tandardizing has become a central feature of social and cultural life in modernity." In *Seeing Like a State*, James Scott's examination of the modern state, he uses the examples of forestry and census-taking to demonstrate how the state simplified landscapes and populations through the natural and social sciences to render the world visible to bureaucrats through abstraction. In theory, this abstraction made people and landscapes easier to manage through a centralized governance structure and in accordance with scientific practices and "fiscal logics." In practice, the reality was a good deal messier. Therefore, central to the project of simplification was the creation of a standard set of measurements—the metric system. For a modern state, like South Africa in the second quarter of the twentieth century, standardization was seen as a way to streamline procedures, regulate behavior, and maximize economic output. This was central to articulating Pholela and COPC. And this is still the case today. As Vincanne Adams writes, "Metrics are technologies of counting, but specifically technologies of counting that form global knowledge." Martha Lampland and Susan Leigh Star, *Standards and Their Stories: How Quantifying, Classifying, and Formalizing Practices Shape Everyday Life* (Ithaca, NY: Cornell University Press, 2009), 10; Geoffrey C. Bowker and Susan Leigh Star, *Sorting Things Out: Classification and Its Consequences* (Cambridge, MA: MIT Press, 2000); James C. Scott, *Seeing Like a State: How Certain Schemes to Improve the Human Condition Have Failed* (New Haven, CT: Yale University Press, 1998); Keith Breckenridge, *Biometric State* (Cambridge:

Cambridge University Press, 2014); Vincanne Adams, *Metrics: What Counts in Global Health* (Durham, NC: Duke University Press, 2016), 6.

9 *Inyanga* is often translated as herbalist. Herbalists make *imithi*, but do not work with the ancestors. The people I work with sometimes call them pharmacists as a way to denote that they know how to make medicines, but they don't have the special connection to the ancestors that *izangoma* (another category of healers) have. As a result, they treat many different illnesses, not just illnesses from ancestors or witchcraft.

10 While much of the background information for these claims came out of conversations with older women in the communities around Pholela, there were hints of residents' misleading answers in health center documents and publications. For example, see 1945 Annual Report, National Archives Repository, Pretoria (SAB), Department of Health files (GES), vol. 1917, ref. 46/32, 38; Cecil Slome, "Community Health in Rural Pholela," in *A Practice of Social Medicine: A South African Team's Experiences in Different African Communities*, ed. Sidney L. Kark and Guy W. Steuart (Edinburgh: E. & S. Livingstone, 1962), 282.

11 "Pholela Centre Provides 'Pilot Plan' for Native Health Schemes" (newspaper article), March 10, 1945, SAB, GES vol. 2704, ref. 2/62.

12 1945 Annual Report, appendices; Kark and Steuart, *A Practice of Social Medicine*, 194; John Cassel, "A Comprehensive Health Program among South African Zulus," in *Health, Culture, and Community: Case Studies of Public Reactions to Health Programs*, ed. Benjamin D. Paul and Walter B. Miller (New York: Russell Sage Foundation, 1955).

13 Biruk defines accuracy as "a true representation of reality, or an individual, or a phenomenon." This is in contrast to precision, which "mandates that data and findings resulting from it must be replicable." This separation is useful in Pholela, where results gathered were precise—they were replicable—but were not always accurate. Crystal Biruk, "Seeing Like a Research Project: Producing 'High-Quality Data' in AIDS Research in Malawi," *Medical Anthropology* 31, no. 4 (2012): 347–66, 353. For analyses of resistance, see James C. Scott, *Weapons of the Weak: Everyday Forms of Peasant Resistance* (New Haven, CT: Yale University Press, 1985); Scott, *Seeing Like a State*. Also see Lampland and Star, *Standards and Their Stories*; Crystal Biruk and Dana Prince, "'Subjects, Participants, Collaborators': Reading Community in Public Health Literature," *International Feminist Journal of Politics* 10, no. 2 (2008): 236–46.

14 Biruk, "Seeing Like a Research Project"; Biruk, *Cooking Data*.

15 See also Martha Lampland, "False Numbers as Formalizing Practices," *Social Studies of Science* 40, no. 3 (2010): 377–404.

16 Sidney L. Kark and Emily Kark, *Promoting Community Health: From Pholela to Jerusalem* (Johannesburg: University of the Witwatersrand Press, 1999), 40.

17 As Kim England writes, "[T]he research encounter is structured by both the researcher and the research participants, and . . . the research, researched *and* researcher might be transformed by the field work experience." Kim V. L. England, "Getting Personal: Reflexivity, Positionality, and Feminist Research," *Professional Geographer* 46, no. 1 (1994): 86.

18   Julie-Kathy Gibson-Graham, "'Stuffed If I Know!': Reflections on Post-Modern Feminist Social Research," *Gender, Place and Culture* 1, no. 2 (1994): 205–24.

19   The idea of reflexivity dates back at least to the 1980s, when feminist scholars began calling for attention to the role of the researcher in the production of knowledge. For example, see Sandra Harding, *Feminism and Methodology: Social Science Issues* (Bloomington: Indiana University Press, 1987); Sandra Harding, *Whose Science? Whose Knowledge?: Thinking from Women's Lives* (Ithaca, NY: Cornell University Press, 1991); Donna J. Haraway, "Situated Knowledges: The Science Question in Feminism and the Privilege of Partial Perspective," *Feminist Studies* 14, no. 3 (1988): 575–99; England, "Getting Personal"; Gillian Rose, "Situating Knowledges: Positionality, Reflexivities and Other Tactics," *Progress in Human Geography* 21, no. 3 (1997): 305–20; Farhana Sultana, "Reflexivity, Positionality and Participatory Ethics: Negotiating Fieldwork Dilemmas in International Research," *ACME: An International E-Journal for Critical Geographies* 6, no. 3 (2007): 374–85.

20   Kobayashi, "Coloring the Field," 76.

21   England, "Getting Personal."

22   The idea of the assemblage draws on the work of Félix Guattari and Giles Deleuze and emerges in conversation with scholars who offer actor-network theory (ANT) as a way to understand human–nonhuman relationships. See endnote 24 in the introduction for more information. Ben Anderson et al., "On Assemblages and Geography," *Dialogues in Human Geography* 2, no. 2 (2012): 184; Gilles Deleuze and Félix Guattari, *Anti-Oedipus* (London: A&C Black, 2004); Gilles Deleuze and Félix Guattari, *A Thousand Plateaus: Capitalism and Schizophrenia*, translated by B. Massumi (Minneapolis: University of Minnesota Press, 1987); Martin Müller, "Assemblages and Actor-Networks: Rethinking Socio-Material Power, Politics and Space," *Geography Compass* 9, no. 1 (2015): 27–41.

23   1945 Annual Report, 32; Letter on water and sanitation to secretary for public health, 1942, SAB, GES vol. 2704, ref. 2/62, ; Slome, "Community Health in Rural Pholela," 288. Residents also often commented on the waste disposal system introduced by the health center.

24   As Kark wrote in the 1945 Annual Report, "Advice is given regarding any new huts or larger homes that are being constructed. Such advise [*sic*] is for the present mainly concerned with increasing the height of the walls and enlarging the window space." 1945 Annual Report, 32.

25   While it is unlikely that the PCHC was fixated on bacteria, they certainly taught about various germs and their role in illness.

26   In the National Library of Medicine's exhibit on Pholela's influence on social medicine, they highlight the importance of the farming cooperative at the Delta Health Center in Mound Bayou, Mississippi. National Library of Medicine, "Community Health: A Model for the World," https://apps.nlm.nih.gov/againsttheodds/exhibit/community_health/model_world.cfm.

27   Marianne de Laet and Annemarie Mol, "The Zimbabwe Bush Pump: Mechanics of a Fluid Technology," *Social Studies of Science* 30, no. 2 (2000): 225–63.

28 Jane Bennett, *Vibrant Matter: A Political Ecology of Things* (Durham, NC: Duke University Press, 2009), 4.

29 Bruno Latour, *Reassembling the Social: An Introduction to Actor-Network-Theory* (Oxford: Oxford University Press, 2005), 107. Emphasis in the original.

30 Sara Ahmed, "Orientations Matter," in *New Materialisms: Ontology, Agency, and Politics*, ed. Diana Coole, 234–57 (Durham, NC: Duke University Press, 2010), 245.

31 Lyn Schumaker, *Africanizing Anthropology: Fieldwork, Networks, and the Making of Cultural Knowledge in Central Africa* (Durham, NC: Duke University Press, 2001), 249.

32 Bruce Braun, "Editorial: Querying Posthumanisms," *Geoforum* 35 (2004): 273.

33 Marilyn Strathern, "Don't Eat Unwashed Lettuce," *American Ethnologist* 33, no. 4 (2006): 532–34, 532.

34 Rose, "Situating Knowledges," 315.

35 Schumaker, *Africanizing Anthropology*, 249.

36 Sandra Harding, "Postcolonial and Feminist Philosophies of Science and Technology: Convergences and Dissonances," *Postcolonial Studies* 12, no. 4 (2009): 401–21, 403.

37 In particular, Sandra Harding's "standpoint theory" and Donna Haraway's "situated knowledges" encourage an understanding of science that starts from the standpoint or the situation of people who are often written out of stories of scientific achievement, namely women and marginalized people, especially those from the Global South. Recently, scholars have brought attention to intersectionality in science studies scholarship. As Banu Subramaniam writes, "The best [feminist science studies] thinkers have used an intersectional idea of gender—locating it in the complexities of race, class, sexuality and nationality." Here Subramaniam is drawing from work that traces to Kimberlee Crenshaw, who coined the term *intersectionality* to highlight the ways in which people with particular intersecting identities—black, poor, queer, women, for example—face multiple axes of discrimination that are different from those who share just one or two of those identities. Wenda K. Bauchspies and Maria Puig de La Bellacasa, "Feminist Science and Technology Studies: A Patchwork of Moving Subjectivities. An Interview with Geoffrey Bowker, Sandra Harding, Anne Marie Mol, Susan Leigh Star and Banu Subramaniam," *Subjectivity* 28, no. 1 (2009): 334–44, 339; Sandra Harding, *The Science Question in Feminism* (Ithaca, NY: Cornell University Press, 1986); Haraway, "Situated Knowledges"; Anne Pollock and Banu Subramaniam, "Resisting Power, Retooling Justice: Promises of Feminist Postcolonial Technosciences," *Science, Technology, and Human Values* 41, no. 6 (2016): 951–66.

38 For example, see Donna J. Haraway, *Simians, Cyborgs, and Women: The Reinvention of Nature* (New York: Routledge, 1991); Donna J. Haraway, *Primate Visions: Gender, Race, and Nature in the World of Modern Science* (New York: Psychology Press, 1989); Donna J. Haraway, *When Species Meet* (Minneapolis: University of Minnesota Press, 2008). Also see Karen Barad for an excellent analysis of the role of scientific apparatuses in the production of scientific knowledge and worlds, *Meeting the Universe Halfway: Quantum Physics and the Entanglement of Matter and Meaning* (Durham, NC: Duke University Press, 2007).

Chapter 3: Nutrition, Science, and Racial Capitalism

1 Sidney L. Kark and Emily Kark, *Promoting Community Health: From Pholela to Jerusalem* (Johannesburg: University of the Witwatersrand Press, 1999).

2 Kark and Kark, *Promoting Community Health*, 45; Cecil Slome, "Community Health in Rural Pholela," in *A Practice of Social Medicine: A South African Team's Experiences in Different African Communities*, ed. Sidney L. Kark and Guy W. Steuart (Edinburgh: E. & S. Livingstone, 1962), 275.

3 Sidney L. Kark, "Migrant Labour and Family Health," in *A Practice of Social Medicine: A South African Team's Experiences in Different African Communities*, ed. Sidney L. Kark and Guy W. Steuart (Edinburgh: E. & S. Livingstone, 1962), 208.

4 One of the most striking things I found when working in the National Archives in Pretoria and the Historical Papers at the University of the Witwatersrand was how many files from the middle of the twentieth century were dedicated to nutrition. Nutrition, especially among Africans, was a national preoccupation, if not an obsession.

5 Chief Native Commissioner of the Cape, "Memorandum on National Health Services," 1945, National Archives Repository, Pretoria (SAB), Secretary of Native Affairs (NTS) vol. 6774, ref. 164/315.

6 As mentioned in chapter 1, the South African Institute of Race Relations is an important, multiracial organization dedicated to the fight for equality.

7 These concerns culminated in the establishment of the National Nutrition Council with the Public Health Amendment Act (Act no. 14) in 1940. Significantly, I found a number of files and pamphlets about nutrition in the South African Institute of Race Relations' files. Filed with academic publications, government reports, speeches, and correspondence, these pamphlets offer a clear signal that concerns over nutrition were central to concerns over equality and justice among some of the government's harshest critics. In South Africa in the 1930s, 1940s, and 1950s, nutrition was politics. For example, see Historical Papers, University of the Witwatersrand, Johannesburg (WHP), South African Institute of Race Relations Papers (SAIRR), part 1 (AD 843/B), 63 and 11. Published sources about nutrition include Henry Gluckman, *Report of the National Health Services Commission on the Provision of an Organized National Health Service for All Sections of the People of the Union of South Africa, 1942–1944* (Pretoria: Government Printer, 1944), 28–30; Eustace Henry Cluver, *Social Medicine* (Johannesburg: Central News Agency), 526; Diana Wylie, *Starving on a Full Stomach: Hunger and the Triumph of Cultural Racism in Modern South Africa* (Charlottesville: University Press of Virginia, 2001).

8 F. W. Fox, "Nutrition and Commonsense: The New Food Knowledge and Some Fallacies," WHP, SAIRR AD 843 B11.3.

9 Fox and Back write: "[R]egarded as the condition of one of the main reserves of labour on which the future prosperity of the Union must partly depend, the problem [of insufficient agricultural production] at once becomes one for urgent attention, too costly to the nation as a whole to be allowed to continue to drift." F. William Fox and Douglas Back, "A Preliminary Survey of the Agricultural

and Nutritional Problems of the Ciskei and Transkeian Territories with Special Reference to Their Bearing on the Recruiting of Labourers for the Gold Mining Industry" (Johannesburg: Unpublished MS, 1943), 308.

10 Fox and Back, "A Preliminary Survey," 1.

11 See Randall Packard's work on the impact of diseases like tuberculosis and malaria on the mining workforce in South Africa. Randall M. Packard, *White Plague, Black Labor: Tuberculosis and the Political Economy of Health and Disease in South Africa* (Berkeley: University of California Press, 1989).

12 A number of scholars have written about South Africa's migrant labor system and its basic assumption that the supply of African laborers was inexhaustible. Dorrit Posel, "How Do Households Work? Migration, the Household and Remittance Behaviour in South Africa," *Social Dynamics* 27, no. 1 (2001): 165–89; Patrick Harries, *Work, Culture, and Identity: Migrant Laborers in Mozambique and South Africa, c. 1860–1910* (Portsmouth, NH: Heinemann, 1994); Alan Jeeves and J. S. Crush, *White Farms, Black Labor: The State and Agrarian Change in Southern Africa, 1910–50* (Portsmouth, NH: James Currey, 1997); Randall M. Packard, "The 'Healthy Reserve' and the 'Dressed Native': Discourses on Black Health and the Language of Legitimation in South Africa," *American Ethnologist* 16, no. 4 (1989): 686–703; Randall M. Packard, "The Invention of the 'Tropical Worker': Medical Research and the Quest for Central African Labor on the South African Gold Mines, 1903–36," *Journal of Southern African Studies* 34, no. 2 (1993): 271–92.

13 Cedric J. Robinson, *Black Marxism: The Making of the Black Radical Tradition* (Chapel Hill: University of North Carolina Press, 2000). Antecedents to the concept of racial capitalism can be found in the work of W. E. B. Du Bois, especially his work on the long-term implications of slavery for the economy globally. W. E. B. Du Bois, *Black Reconstruction in America: Toward a History of the Part Which Black Folk Played in the Attempt to Reconstruct Democracy in America, 1860–1880* (London: Routledge, 2017).

14 Robin D. G. Kelley, "What Did Cedric Robinson Mean by Racial Capitalism?," *Boston Review*, January 12, 2017.

15 Kelley, "What Did Cedric Robinson Mean by Racial Capitalism?"

16 Walter Rodney, *How Europe Underdeveloped Africa* (Washington, DC: Howard University Press, 1972).

17 While global, the relationships around both race and class that make up racial capitalism make particularly strong impressions in settler states. South Africa, especially under apartheid, offers one of the most obvious and striking examples of this, as living spaces were strictly segregated, black workers were inputs into a system of white profit, and rural African homelands were labor reserves. By the second quarter of the twentieth century, the imbrications of racism and capitalism were so strong that they shaped all government policy, from housing to labor to nutrition and health. This is why any discussion of political economy in South Africa is necessarily a discussion about racial capitalism. For more on southern and South Africa specifically, see Harries, *Work, Culture, and Identity*; Saul Dubow, *Racial Segregation and the Origins of Apartheid in South Africa, 1919–36* (Basingstoke,

UK: Palgrave Macmillan, 1989); Anthony W. Marx, *Making Race and Nation: A Comparison of South Africa, the United States, and Brazil* (Cambridge: Cambridge University Press, 1998). For an understanding of racial capitalism in South Africa postapartheid and in the era of globalization, see Gillian Patricia Hart, *Disabling Globalization: Places of Power in Post-Apartheid South Africa* (Berkeley: University of California Press, 2002).

18 Harold Wolpe, "Capitalism and Cheap Labour-Power in South Africa: From Segregation to Apartheid," *Economy and Society* 1, no. 4 (1972): 425–56, 454.

19 In the end, the mining companies found another way to solve their labor woes—they recruited workers from neighboring countries, thereby making their labor supply appear almost endless. With time and changes in immigration policies, however, even this was not enough. For an example of what this meant in terms of health, see Packard, "The Invention of the 'Tropical Worker.'"

20 Elias Mandala, "Feeding and Fleecing the Native: How the Nyasaland Transport System Distorted a New Food Market, 1890s–1920s," *Journal of Southern African Studies* 32, no. 3 (2006): 503–24.

21 A report entitled "Health Policy in Relation to Nutrition Needs" revealed that this mismatch between food production and nutritional needs was a countrywide phenomenon. While the data were scattershot and the population-scale analysis covered over inequities within South Africa, the study revealed two things: First, the data focused attention on the relationships between agriculture and nutrition, and second, data revealed that South Africa was not even close to producing enough "protective" foods for its population. (It did, however, produce plenty of calorie-dense and nutritionally inferior foods like maize.) Even if the economic question could be settled, agricultural production was insufficient for the needs of the population. D. G. Haylett, "Food Resources of the Union in Relation to the Nutritional Requirements of the Population," WHP, SAIRR AD 843-RJ, Na14, File 1.

22 While in hindsight what amounted to a call for higher wages might seem rather obvious, it was not at that time. After all, Fox and Back's was a study commissioned by the mining industry, the very group that would have to pay those higher wages.

23 Haylett, "Food Resources of the Union," 5.

24 Kenneth J. Carpenter, "A Short History of Nutritional Science: Part 3 (1912–1944)," *Journal of Nutrition* 133, no. 10 (2003): 3023–32, 3031.

25 Carpenter, "A Short History of Nutritional Science: Part 3"; Kenneth J. Carpenter, "A Short History of Nutritional Science: Part 4 (1945–1985)," *Journal of Nutrition* 133, no. 11 (2003): 3331–42.

26 Letter from secretary for public health to the secretary for native affairs, October 13, 1942, SAB NTS 7886 115/336(6).

27 Haylett, "Food Resources of the Union."

28 *Coloured* is a racial classification in South Africa that refers to people who most often have a mix of African and European ancestry. Cluver, *Social Medicine*, 526.

29 For example, see the South African Institute of Race Relations (SAIRR) Papers from the University of the Witwatersrand's Historical Papers (WHP) on nu-

trition, which include many of the government's policies on mine rations and school lunches, as well as the medical science that underpinned those policies. WHP, SAIRR, part I (AD 843/B), 63.

30 Julie Guthman, "Introducing Critical Nutrition: A Special Issue on Dietary Advice and Its Discontents," *Gastronomica* 14, no. 3 (2014): 1–4; Allison Hayes-Conroy and Jessica Hayes-Conroy, "Taking Back Taste: Feminism, Food and Visceral Politics," *Gender, Place and Culture* 15, no. 5 (2008): 461–73; Aya H. Kimura et al., "Nutrition as a Project," *Gastronomica: The Journal of Critical Food Studies* 14, no. 3 (2014): 34–45.

31 Wylie, *Starving on a Full Stomach*. In their edited volume *Knowing Nature*, Mara Goldman, Paul Nadasdy, and Matthew Turner seek to combine critical understandings of the production, circulation, and application of scientific knowledge in an effort to understand all aspects of environmental science through a combination of science studies and political ecology. While not directly relevant, this volume has been deeply important for my thinking and echoes many of the lessons of Wylie's book. Mara J. Goldman, Paul Nadasdy, and Matthew D. Turner, *Knowing Nature: Conversations at the Intersection of Political Ecology and Science Studies* (Chicago: University of Chicago Press, 2011).

32 Wylie, *Starving on a Full Stomach*, 239.

33 A number of other scholars have shown that eating nutritiously has been linked to being good, responsible citizens, valuable subjects of a nation, and participants in an economy. For example, see Kimura et al., "Nutrition as a Project."

34 Of course, South Africa is not the only place where race and nutrition were and are entangled. For example, in Nik Heynen's work on the Black Panthers' Food Not Bombs program, he explains that even though the Panthers established the country's first free breakfast program for children in 1969—the predecessor to the national school lunch program—their history gets lost in a thick web of expectations that see black people as culturally inferior when it comes to food and nutrition. In the United States, as well as in South Africa, the social worlds of racial capitalism shape everything from official policy to science to memory to food and nutrition. Nik Heynen, "Bending the Bars of Empire from Every Ghetto for Survival: The Black Panther Party's Radical Antihunger Politics of Social Reproduction and Scale," *Annals of the Association of American Geographers* 99, no. 2 (2009): 406–22.

35 PCHC Monthly Reports, SAB, Department of Health files (GES), LEER vol. 2704, ref. 2/62.

36 In talking with people about their vegetable gardens in the past and today, they talk about the difficulty of growing some vegetables like tomatoes and not others like beans, often citing the soil, environment, or climate as the reason particular foods would not grow.

37 1945 Annual Report, SAB, GES, vol. 1917, ref. 46/32, 32; John Cassel, "A Comprehensive Health Program among South African Zulus," in *Health, Culture, and Community: Case Studies of Public Reactions to Health Programs*, ed. Benjamin D. Paul and Walter B. Miller (New York: Russell Sage Foundation, 1955).

38   Sidney L. Kark and Guy W. Steuart, *A Practice of Social Medicine: A South African Team's Experiences in Different African Communities* (Edinburgh: E. & S. Livingstone, 1962).

39   1945 Annual Report; Sidney L. Kark, *The Practice of Community-Oriented Primary Health Care* (New York: Appleton-Century-Crofts, 1981).

40   PCHC Monthly Report, February 5, 1941, SAB, GES vol. 2704, ref. 2-62. In their memoir, the Karks discuss the logic behind the demonstration gardens and the food prescriptions. Kark and Kark, *Promoting Community Health*, 49.

41   1945 Annual Report, 20–21, 50–51.

42   Kark, *The Practice of Community-Oriented Primary Health Care*, 209; Sidney L. Kark and Emily Kark, "Epidemiological Considerations of Malnutrition in Rural African School Children," in *A Practice of Social Medicine: A South African Team's Experiences in Different African Communities*, ed. Sidney L. Kark and Guy W. Steuart (Edinburgh: E. & S. Livingstone, 1962).

43   Residents often commented on the health center's demonstration garden and what they learned there. 1945 Annual Report, 16–17; Cassel, "A Comprehensive Health Program among South African Zulus," 26; Slome, "Community Health in Rural Pholela," 279.

44   Slome, "Community Health in Rural Pholela," 278–79.

45   Sidney L. Kark and John Cassel, "The Pholela Health Centre: A Progress Report," *South African Medical Journal* 26, no. 6 (1952): 132. See also Cassel, "A Comprehensive Health Program among South African Zulus," 26.

46   Kark, *The Practice of Community-Oriented Primary Health Care*, 238.

47   1950 Annual Report, SAB, GES, vol. 1917, ref. 46/32, 28.

48   Slome, "Community Health in Rural Pholela," 277.

49   Slome, "Community Health in Rural Pholela," 278.

50   Cassel, "A Comprehensive Health Program among South African Zulus"; Kark and Kark, *Promoting Community Health*; Kark, *The Practice of Community-Oriented Primary Health Care*; Kark and Steuart, *A Practice of Social Medicine*; Slome, "Community Health in Rural Pholela."

51   Carpenter, "A Short History of Nutritional Science: Part 4."

52   For information on eggs, see Elizabeth Applegate, "Introduction: Nutritional and Functional Roles of Eggs in the Diet," *Journal of the American College of Nutrition* 19, supp. 5 (2000): 495S–98S.

53   Cassel, "A Comprehensive Health Program among South African Zulus," 27.

54   Cassel, "A Comprehensive Health Program among South African Zulus."

55   Annual Reports, SAB, GES 1917; Kark, *The Practice of Community-Oriented Primary Health Care*, 228; Kark and Kark, *Promoting Community Health*, 48.

56   Kark, "A Practice of Social Medicine," 206.

57   See documents from SAB, GES 1917; SAB, GES 2704; Gluckman, *Report of the National Health Services Commission*, 26.

58   Cassel, "A Comprehensive Health Program among South African Zulus," 28–29.

59   Cassel, "A Comprehensive Health Program among South African Zulus"; Slome, "Community Health in Rural Pholela."

60 Slome, "Community Health in Rural Pholela," 279. The markets that developed around residents' gardens never developed around milk because of the relationships between cows and ancestors for residents and because of the relative scarcity of cows.

61 Of course, Pholela was not unique in this respect; the inadequate available land was the result of a national land tenure system in which the majority African population was restricted to a small minority of the land.

62 For a more in-depth analysis of food taboos, see Abigail H. Neely, "Hlonipha and Health," *Africa*, 91, vol. 3 (2021).

63 A number of scholars have written on intra-household eating patterns, often noting that men are to be served first, followed by older women, children, and then other women. When I asked people about food-serving protocols, this is often what I heard. In practice, however, things are a good bit more complicated, both because those preparing food often snack as they go and because mealtimes are seldom routinized. For example, in their work on hunger in Pholela, the health center found that girls suffered less malnutrition than boys because of the role they played in the kitchen. And in her ethnography on Pondoland, just to the west of Pholela, Monica Wilson found that mealtimes were unpredictable enough that in practice, the strict hierarchy of serving and eating was a good bit more complicated. The result was that it was hard to predict who might suffer from malnutrition due to home consumption. This was especially true for foods that did not have taboos or consumption restrictions applied to them. Once a crisis like a famine hits a community, however, food consumption tends to follow hierarchies. As Megan Vaughan details in her examination of the 1949 famine in Nyasaland, the impact of famine—starvation—was not felt equally across the population. Kark and Kark, *Promoting Community Health*; Monica Wilson, *Reaction to Conquest: Effects of Contact with Europeans on the Pondo of South Africa* (London: Oxford University Press, 1936); Megan Vaughan, *The Story of an African Famine: Gender and Famine in Twentieth-Century Malawi* (New York: Cambridge University Press, 1987).

64 Slome, "Community Health in Rural Pholela," 281. For a more complete explanation, see Kark, *The Practice of Community-Oriented Primary Health Care*, 239–40.

65 Kark, *The Practice of Community-Oriented Primary Health Care*, 201.

66 Richard A. Schroeder, *Shady Practices: Agroforestry and Gender Politics in the Gambia* (Berkeley: University of California Press, 1999); Matthew Turner, "Drought, Domestic Budgeting and Wealth Distribution in Sahelian Households," *Development and Change* 31, no. 5 (2000): 1009–35.

67 The most well known proponent of the concept of structural violence is Paul Farmer. He argues that ill health in Haiti is rooted in poverty and uneven global political-economic structures that have a detrimental impact on individual bodies through disease, violence, and inadequate health care. He uses this concept to explain the devastating health impacts of global political-economic structures as manifest in development aid and official policies. One particularly valuable aspect of this work is that it includes the role that poverty has in producing illness as

well as the impact of underfunded health care systems. Paul Farmer, "On Suffering and Structural Violence: A View from Below," *Daedalus* 25, no. 1 (1996): 261–83; Paul Farmer, *Infections and Inequalities: The Modern Plagues* (Berkeley: University of California Press, 1999); Paul Farmer, *Pathologies of Power: Health, Human Rights, and the New War on the Poor* (Berkeley: University of California Press, 2005); Paul Farmer, *AIDS and Accusation: Haiti and the Geography of Blame*, rev. ed. (Berkeley: University of California Press, 2006); Paul Farmer et al., "An Anthropology of Structural Violence 1," *Current Anthropology* 45, no. 3 (2004): 305–25; Seth Holmes, *Fresh Fruit, Broken Bodies: Migrant Farmworkers in the United States* (Berkeley: University of California Press, 2013); Nancy Scheper-Hughes, *Death without Weeping: The Violence of Everyday Life in Brazil* (Berkeley: University of California Press, 1993).

68 For example, see Brian King, "Political Ecologies of Health," *Progress in Human Geography* 34, no. 1 (2010): 38–55; Brian King, "Spatialising Livelihoods: Resource Access and Livelihood Spaces in South Africa," *Transactions of the Institute of British Geographers* 36, no. 2 (2011): 297–313.

69 Julie Guthman, "Opening Up the Black Box of the Body in Geographical Obesity Research: Toward a Critical Political Ecology of Fat," *Annals of the Association of American Geographers* 102, no. 5 (2012): 951–57; Julie Guthman, *Weighing In: Obesity, Food Justice, and the Limits of Capitalism* (Berkeley: University of California Press, 2011); Abigail H. Neely, "Internal Ecologies and the Limits of Local Biologies: A Political Ecology of Tuberculosis in the Time of AIDS," *Annals of the Association of American Geographers* 105, no. 4 (2015): 791–805.

70 I take great inspiration from Becky Mansfield's work on childbirth, in which she outlines an approach that understands health as a "biosocial" practice and process. Becky Mansfield, "Health as a Nature-Society Question," *Environment and Planning A* 40 (2008): 1015–19; Becky Mansfield, "The Social Nature of Natural Childbirth," *Social Science and Medicine* 66, no. 5 (2008): 1084–94; Becky Mansfield, "Environmental Health as Biosecurity: 'Seafood Choices,' Risk, and the Pregnant Woman as Threshold," *Annals of the Association of American Geographers* 102, no. 5 (2012): 969–76.

In addition to political ecologies of health, environmental justice literature ties bodies to landscapes. For these scholars, racial capitalism profoundly shapes the environments in which people live. This means that poor, brown people tend to live in more toxic, less healthy environments. As a result, poor people disproportionately suffer the negative effects of the environments in which they live. The effects of these environments then manifest in their bodies. The corollary is also true. As Julie Guthman argues in her book on obesity in America, people who live in "healthy" environments ("leptogenic" in her words) and have access to fresh food they can afford have lower rates of obesity and the diseases that correlate with it. Nikolas C. Heynen, "The Scalar Production of Injustice within the Urban Forest," *Antipode* 35, no. 5 (2003): 980–98; Ryan Holifield, "Defining Environmental Justice and Environmental Racism," *Urban Geography* 22, no. 1 (2001): 78–90; Laura Pulido, "Rethinking Environmental Racism: White Privilege and Urban Development in Southern California," *Annals of the Association of American Geogra-*

phers 90, no. 1 (2000): 12–40; Erik Swyngedouw and Nikolas C. Heynen, "Urban Political Ecology, Justice and the Politics of Scale," *Antipode* 35, no. 5 (2003): 898–918; Laura Pulido, *Black, Brown, Yellow, and Left: Radical Activism in Los Angeles* (Berkeley: University of California Press, 2006); Guthman, *Weighing In*.

71 Political ecologists and environmental historians have long been interested in questions about erosion. For example, see Piers M. Blaikie, H. C. Brookfield, *Land Degradation and Society* (New York: Methuen, 1987); Timothy Forsyth, "Mountain Myths Revisited: Integrating Natural and Social Environmental Science," *Mountain Research and Development* 18, no. 2 (1998): 107–16; Kate Showers, *Imperial Gullies: Soil Erosion and Conservation in Lesotho* (Athens: Ohio University Press, 2005).

72 I must thank Julie Guthman for pointing out the parallels between Blaikie and Brookfield's work and that of the PCHC. Blaikie and Brookfield, *Land Degradation and Society*.

73 This is a term I developed in a piece on TB and HIV. Neely, "Internal Ecologies and the Limits of Local Biologies."

74 I use the idea of scale here in recognition of the fact that scale is socially constructed, per chapter 2.

75 In spite of all of the reports about these broad problems, little was done to improve the lives of poor Africans on a national level.

76 In *Starving on a Full Stomach*, Diana Wylie writes of the importance for African diets of South Africa's regulatory body setting the price of foods, moderating production, and addressing overproduction in the post–World War II era. Wylie, *Starving on a Full Stomach*, 205.

77 By the late 1940s, however, the government came to see the redistributive logics of this practice as a threat. Indeed, it was the practice of giving out food parcels for *free* as prescriptions that prompted the apartheid government to investigate Sidney Kark as a communist in the 1950s (in spite of the fact that he had no ties to the prominent Communist Party in South Africa). Investigations like these would eventually lead Kark, and many of his colleagues, to leave South Africa. Kark and Kark, *Promoting Community Health*, viii.

78 This is the central lesson of structural violence.

79 Karen Barad, *Meeting the Universe Halfway: Quantum Physics and the Entanglement of Matter and Meaning* (Durham, NC: Duke University Press, 2007), 65.

80 In many senses, these limitations are an old story, often told in the accounts of political ecologists who point out that the restrictions of political economy do more to constrain behavior and damage environments than the peasants who are so often blamed for it.

Chapter 4: Witchcraft and the Limits of Social Medicine

1 Sidney L. Kark and Guy W. Steuart, *A Practice of Social Medicine: A South African Team's Experiences in Different African Communities* (Edinburgh: E. & S. Livingstone, 1962), 286.

2 As Stacey Langwick points out, David Bloor, one of the founders of SSK (the so-

ciology of scientific knowledge), first called for symmetry in analysis in 1976, and many other scholars have followed suit, including Bruno Latour. For example, see David Bloor, *Knowledge and Social Imagery* (Chicago: University of Chicago Press, 1991); Michel Callon and Bruno Latour, "Don't Throw the Baby Out with the Bath School! A Reply to Collins and Yearley," *Science as Practice and Culture* 343 (1992): 368; Stacey Ann Langwick, *Bodies, Politics, and African Healing: The Matter of Maladies in Tanzania* (Bloomington: Indiana University Press, 2011).

3 Langwick, *Bodies, Politics, and African Healing*, 34.

4 By this I mean that many scholars have argued that witchcraft accusations help to regulate antisocial behavior as people prefer to avoid conflict so that it will not be possible for them to be implicated in witchcraft. Likewise, if people do behave outside of the expected norms, witchcraft accusations help to force a modification of behavior to better align with the expectations of the group. For example, see Adam Ashforth, *Madumo: A Man Bewitched* (Chicago: University of Chicago Press, 2000); Adam Ashforth, *Witchcraft, Violence, and Democracy in South Africa* (Chicago: University of Chicago Press, 2005); Harriet Ngubane, *Body and Mind in Zulu Medicine: An Ethnography of Health and Disease in Nyuswa-Zulu Thought and Practice* (London: Academic Press, 1977); Isak A. Niehaus, Eliazaar Mohlala, and Kally Shokane, *Witchcraft, Power, and Politics: Exploring the Occult in the South African Lowveld* (London: Pluto, 2001).

5 Ashforth, *Witchcraft, Violence, and Democracy in South Africa*.

6 Steven Feierman and John Janzen, along with several other scholars, have understood witchcraft as one category of illness in a wider portfolio of illness for Bantu peoples of southern and eastern Africa. This is important work, as it is some of the earliest scholarship to understand health and healing from the perspective of African peoples. At the same time, these scholars understand health in this way through a framework of solely human social life. So, while it is an important way to understand health from Pholela, it also has some of the same limitations as the other scholarship on witchcraft. Steven Feierman, "Struggles for Control: The Social Roots of Health and Healing in Modern Africa," *African Studies Review* 28, nos. 2–3 (1985): 73–147; Steven Feierman, "Explaining Uncertainty in the Medical World of Ghaambo," *Bulletin of the History of Medicine* 74 (2000): 317–44; Steven Feierman and John M. Janzen, eds., *The Social Basis of Health and Healing in Africa* (Berkeley: University of California Press, 1992); John M. Janzen, "Therapy Management: Concept, Reality, Process," *Medical Anthropology Quarterly* 1, no. 1 (1987): 68–84; John M. Janzen, *Ngoma: Discourses of Healing in Central and Southern Africa* (Berkeley: University of California Press, 1992).

7 It is important to note that these two statistics are for different populations. As I explained in chapter 1, each year the Designated Area expanded, incorporating more and more households, and therefore the number of households surveyed also expanded. As a result, one must be cautious in making comparisons between the two, though doing so was part of the PCHC's practice. That said, it is clear that the trend for tuberculosis not only diverged from the trend of other illnesses in Pholela, but that it did so markedly. John Cassel, "A Comprehensive Health Program among South African Zulus," in *Health, Culture, and Community; Case*

Studies of Public Reactions to Health Programs, ed. Benjamin D. Paul and Walter B. Miller (New York: Russell Sage Foundation, 1955), 29; Cecil Slome, "Community Health in Rural Pholela," in *A Practice of Social Medicine: A South African Team's Experiences in Different African Communities*, ed. Sidney L. Kark and Guy W. Steuart, 284–85 (Edinburgh: E. & S. Livingstone, 1962).

8 The Karks did not name the people in their write-up in the annual report. I've added names in an effort to make the analysis clearer.

9 1944 Annual Report, National Archives Repository, Pretoria (SAB), Department of Health files (GES), vol. 1917, ref. 46/32, 49.

10 There is no breakdown of tuberculosis statistics for "good" versus "bad" households. Given that 25 percent of households had at least one member with tuberculosis and that 89 percent of households kept vegetable gardens (i.e., participated in health center programs and were therefore "good"), it seems reasonable to assume that even "good" households had cases of tuberculosis. For tuberculosis statistics, see Cassel, "A Comprehensive Health Program among South African Zulus," 29; Sidney L. Kark, *The Practice of Community-Oriented Primary Health Care* (New York: Appleton-Century-Crofts, 1981), 237–38; Sidney L. Kark and John Cassel, "The Pholela Health Centre: A Progress Report," *South African Medical Journal* 26, no. 6 (1952): 132; Slome, "Community Health in Rural Pholela," 279, 84–85. For garden statistics, see PCHC annual reports, SAB, GES, vol. 1917, ref. 46/32.

11 As Eustice Cluver, social medicine expert of the time and later a colleague of the Karks, wrote, "Tuberculosis is so closely related to the social structure of the community that its prevalence is often used as a standard by which the social adequacy of a community can be measured." Eustace Henry Cluver, *Social Medicine* (Johannesburg: Central News Agency, 1951), 271.

12 As the doctors wrote in the conclusion of their case summary: "[O]f importance is the approach to the problem—the case of active tuberculosis being regarded as the expression of a set of social, cultural and economic conditions of the family, each of which has to be treated: —the social by improving accommodation (especially sleeping accommodation) and personal habits (cleanliness, sanitation); the cultural by aiming to re-educate the family, a) in its concept of disease and b) getting the younger children to school; economic by increasing production of food stuffs with the use of more advanced methods (e.g., anti-soil erosion measures, manufacture of humus from household and animal refuse), and by encouraging and assisting the three youths of the family to find employment which will bring in some very necessary cash." 1944 Annual Report, 52.

13 I take this story from a chapter that John Cassel wrote. Cassel does not give the woman a name. As with the previous story, I have added a name here to help locate the reader in the story as I mobilize it in a later, rather complicated theoretical argument. John Cassel, "Cultural Factors in the Interpretation of Illness," in *A Practice of Social Medicine: A South African Team's Experiences in Different African Communities*, ed. Sidney L. Kark and Guy W. Steuart (Edinburgh: E. & S. Livingstone, 1962).

14 A person's father, uncles, husband, and brothers are often key decision makers within health and healing. The health center staff often complained about this practice. Janzen, "Therapy Management."

15 A number of health center staff commented on idliso. I also conducted several interviews with residents, community health workers, and izangoma about idliso and tuberculosis. Finally, Harriet Ngubane writes about idliso in her ethnography about health and healing, as does Adam Ashforth. Slome, "Community Health in Rural Pholela," 284–85; Cassel, "A Comprehensive Health Program among South African Zulus"; Cassel, "Cultural Factors in the Interpretation of Illness"; Ngubane, *Body and Mind in Zulu Medicine*; Ashforth, *Madumo*.

16 Cassel, "A Comprehensive Health Program among South African Zulus," 31.

17 In conversations with izangoma between 2008 and 2016, they told me that it is possible for people to have idliso and tuberculosis. When I asked, residents explained that this was not new. If this is the case, they explained that the person should be treated for one illness, complete the treatment, and then be treated for the second. I suspect that in practice there is a good deal more treatment overlap. I get into this more later.

18 I go into much more detail about this idea in an article. Abigail H. Neely, "Internal Ecologies and the Limits of Local Biologies: A Political Ecology of Tuberculosis in the Time of AIDS," *Annals of the Association of American Geographers* 105, no. 4 (2015): 791–805.

19 This is the process described by Feierman and Janzen and by many people I talked to. As detailed in the introduction, however, reality is often messier than this straightforward, idealized trial-and-error process. Stacey Langwick examines this in her piece on patients accessing multiple kinds of healing in a Tanzanian hospital. To a certain extent, both of these approaches were likely at work in this case. Khanyisile went to the health center once it was clear that the efforts of the inyanga were not working, but it is also likely that she continued to access treatment from multiple healers at once. Feierman, "Explaining Uncertainty in the Medical World of Ghaambo"; John M. Janzen and William Arkinstall, *The Quest for Therapy in Lower Zaire* (Berkeley: University of California Press, 1978); Stacey A. Langwick, "Articulate(d) Bodies: Traditional Medicine in a Tanzanian Hospital," *American Ethnologist* 35, no. 3 (2008): 428–39.

20 To his credit, Cassel recognized this when he reflected on the case. He wrote, "By suggesting that the daughter had started the disease process in this family, the doctor in effect had accused the daughter of possessing the power to spread disease. In this community only sorcerers and witches are recognized as having that power." Cassel, "A Comprehensive Health Program among South African Zulus," 33.

21 The "not yet" part is significant in its aspirational quality as well as its call for personal responsibility under the guise of self-help; Dr. Slome envisioned a future in which Pholela's residents *would be* educated and therefore healthier.

22 Cassel says this directly in his write-up of the case. Cassel, "A Comprehensive Health Program among South African Zulus."

23 Diana Wylie, *Starving on a Full Stomach: Hunger and the Triumph of Cultural Racism in Modern South Africa* (Charlottesville: University Press of Virginia, 2001).

24 Cassel, "A Comprehensive Health Program among South African Zulus," 33–34.

25 According to health center statistics, the incidence of tuberculosis actually increased after the introduction of antibiotics, which were available in Pholela early on. This is different from what one would expect to see, given that antibiotics are the only cure for TB. As a result, it seems possible that the shift to antibiotics as the primary way to treat tuberculosis had a negative effect on tuberculosis rates. In other words, perhaps the holistic approach originally applied was more effective. Given that health center extension work remained consistent through the 1950s, however, I do not think the difference in approach was likely as striking as it appears in the stories presented here.

26 For another example of a confounding TB case, see Cassel, "Cultural Factors in the Interpretation of Illness."

27 1944 Annual Report; Cassel, "A Comprehensive Health Program among South African Zulus."

28 Langwick, *Bodies, Politics, and African Healing*; Abigail H. Neely, "Worlds in a Bottle: An Object-Centered Ethnography for Global Health," *Medicine Anthropology Theory* 6, no. 4 (2019): 127–41; Annemarie Mol, "A Reader's Guide to the 'Ontological Turn'—Part 4," *Somatosphere: Science, Medicine, and Anthropology*, March 19, 2014, http://somatosphere.net/2014/a-readers-guide-to-the-ontological-turn-part-4.html/.

29 I draw inspiration from the work of Eduardo Viveiros de Castro, but with a bit of both caution and skepticism. His work is about thinking with, or allowing to think as, animals. This is inspiring because it offers possibilities for ontological multiplicity. At the same time, given the history of equating peoples of African descent with animals and understanding Africans and other nonwhite peoples as less than human, the application of this work requires both caution and care. With that, I find de Castro's idea of "perspectives" helpful in thinking through witchcraft. In his work in the Amazon, and as a key contributor to the scholarship of the ontological turn, he writes about the different perspectives pigs and people have, asserting that differences in "perspectives" are ontological, rather than epistemological. He writes, "[a]nimals see in the *same* way as we do *different* things." In other words, perspectives are about ontological difference, rather than about dissimilarities in how various groups see, understand, or know the same world; they are differences in worlds, not differences in ideas. I think that extending this lesson to different groups of people highlights the importance of recognizing difference as ontological, rather than as cultural or social. In addition, de Castro posits that these different worlds are not all open to everyone; pigs and people cannot necessarily inhabit one another's realities, at least not on their own terms. For understanding the specifics of social medicine, its possibilities, and its limitations in Pholela, this acknowledgment that worlds are not accessible to everyone—that ontological multiplicity is not intelligible to all—is important. Eduardo Viveiros de Castro, "Cosmological Deixis and Amerindian Perspectivism,"

Journal of the Royal Anthropological Institute (1998): 478; Eduardo Batalha Viveiros de Castro, "Exchanging Perspectives: The Transformation of Objects into Subjects in Amerindian Ontologies," *Common Knowledge* 10, no. 3 (2004): 463–84.

While I have found de Castro's work helpful to think with, it is Pholela's residents who really taught me about ontological multiplicity. Indigenous and Native scholars have been critical of the co-optation of indigenous knowledge both within and outside of the academy. This is particularly well explained in Zoe Todd's article, "An Indigenous Feminist's Take on the Ontological Turn," where she asserts that many of the insights of the ontological turn, posthumanism, cosmopolitics, and so on are built on the backs, stories, lives, and articulations of non-European thinkers and people, with very little attribution to those thinkers and people. In other words, the theoretical advances of people situated at European and Anglo-American institutions and of European descent are rooted in the knowledge of indigenous people at least as much as in Enlightenment philosophical traditions. In addition, in Todd's piece, many important connections are made to the relationships between disciplines like anthropology and colonialism and between higher education and the exploitation of marginalized people. For my purposes, however, the assertion that indigenous people and scholars have always "taken seriously" other worlds, recognizing their claims to reality and therefore their challenge to things like science is particularly important. For while this book might draw from theoretical currents focusing on relational ontologies, Pholela's residents, like the people Todd writes about, have long known that there are multiple worlds, and their lives, experiences, stories, and worlds form the basis for the analysis here. Zoe Todd, "An Indigenous Feminist's Take on the Ontological Turn: 'Ontology' Is Just Another Word for Colonialism," *Journal of Historical Sociology* 29, no. 1 (2016): 4–22.

30 Two important analytics for understanding these relationships are actor-networks and assemblages. As explained in the introduction, two important scholars of these approaches are Bruno Latour (ANT) and Gilles Deleuze (assemblages). Bruno Latour, *Reassembling the Social: An Introduction to Actor-Network-Theory* (Oxford: Oxford University Press, 2005); Bruno Latour, *We Have Never Been Modern* (Cambridge, MA: Harvard University Press, 2012); Gilles Deleuze and Félix Guattari, *Anti-Oedipus* (London: A&C Black, 2004); Gilles Deleuze and Félix Guattari, *A Thousand Plateaus: Capitalism and Schizophrenia*, translated by B. Massumi (Minneapolis: University of Minnesota Press, 1987).

31 The idea of taking these things seriously is a key concept these days. There are a number of lineages for this approach, from the ontological turn in anthropology to scholars interested in questions of decolonization and indigenous life, to scholars with a long-term commitment to ethnography. Whatever the lineage, it is an important research and analytical commitment as it maintains a focus on the lives and experiences of research subjects. I offer more detail on this in the introduction.

32 I learned about imithi and idliso both through the work of the PCHC doctors and through numerous conversations with residents and healers in Pholela today.

33 These "muthi markets" are often referred to today as the "Zulu chemist," or pharmacist in American English.

34 Organizations like the Center for Scientific and Industrial Research (CSIR) in South Africa have conducted research on Zulu medicinal plants to see if they have healing properties. The trouble with testing according to the scientific method is that it screens for efficacy in terms of biomedical diseases and then measures that efficacy in scientific terms. In other words, it's the ingredients and their quantities that matter, not the umthakathi or the ancestors. While this surely accounts for some efficacy, as the rest of the explanation in the text attests, it does not fully grasp all aspects of how the umuthi works. For an account of what happens when plants used in traditional medicine get taken up by biomedicine, bioprospecting, and pharmaceuticals, see Laura A. Foster, *Reinventing Hoodia: Peoples, Plants, and Patents in South Africa* (Seattle: University of Washington Press, 2017).

35 Susan Craddock writes about product development partnerships, groups of individuals and institutions representing for-profit pharmaceutical corporations, individuals, and nongovernmental organizations that have come together in search of a vaccine for one of the world's most devastating diseases for the poor: tuberculosis, and the pharmacological products they make. In her analysis, Craddock reveals that by divorcing product from profit, these PDPs developed a very different kind of drug. Significantly, these drugs were not only different because of the chemicals that made them up, but also because of the social and political-economic relationships through which they were produced. Susan Craddock, *Compound Solutions: Pharmaceutical Alternatives for Global Health* (Minneapolis: University of Minnesota Press, 2017).

36 The production of imithi in Pholela was not unique. For example, Monica Wilson described in detail the production of healing imithi in Pondoland in the 1930s. She points out that the way a treatment was given mattered. Wilson offers the story of a healer who was well known for her ability to treat infertility. When she gave a patient an umuthi, she told her to take it in the morning and evening for a number of months while crossing her hands. This last part—the crossing of the hands—"was an essential part of the cure." If the patient did not cross her hands while taking the imithi, it would not work. As Wilson writes, "[T]he material element is not in itself sufficient," and this "is shown by the insistence of those who have a knowledge of medicines, that they must be used in a particular way." She goes on to explain that a stolen umuthi will only work if a person knows how to use it; its effectiveness is predicated on this knowledge. Likewise, Steven Feierman points out that for the Shambaa of present-day Tanzania, the healer is as essential to the efficacy of the imithi as the individual ingredients that make it up and the way it is used. Monica Wilson, *Reaction to Conquest: Effects of Contact with Europeans on the Pondo of South Africa* (London: Oxford University Press, 1936), 296, 306. Also see Feierman, "Struggles for Control."

37 Mol writes, "It is possible to say that in practices objects are *enacted*. This suggests that activities take place—but leaves actors vague. It also suggests that in the act, and only then and there, something *is*—being enacted." Annemarie Mol, *The Body*

Multiple: Ontology in Medical Practice (Durham, NC: Duke University Press, 2002), 32–33.

38 I invoke Karen Barad with the idea of matter and meaning. Karen Barad, "Post-humanist Performativity: Toward an Understanding of How Matter Comes to Matter," *Signs* 28, no. 3 (2003): 801–31; Karen Barad, *Meeting the Universe Halfway: Quantum Physics and the Entanglement of Matter and Meaning* (Durham, NC: Duke University Press, 2007).

39 I have found the work of Karen Barad particularly generative for my thinking, especially her concept of the phenomenon. Phenomena emerge from entanglements that result from the relationships among phenomena, and more basically from all relationships. With the phenomenon, Barad explores "matter and meaning," things and ideas. The use of "and" here is significant; it indicates a relational approach, rather than an oppositional approach. For my purposes, phenomena are the specific entanglements of matter and meaning that make up illness and wellness. Understanding phenomena, which are entanglements, as primary ontological units is what distinguishes feminist science studies from ANT and assemblage theory. In both ANT and assemblage theory, individuals remain even as they are constantly shaped and reshaped by other individuals. For feminist scholars, relationships are constitutional and there are no individuals. This is important in thinking about how witchcraft works, shifting the focus from individual elements to the phenomenon of the disease. Barad, *Meeting the Universe Halfway*, 141. I offer a more complete explanation of this in Abigail H. Neely, "Entangled Agencies: Rethinking Causality and Health in Political-Ecology," *Environment and Planning E: Nature and Space* (2020), https://doi.org/10.1177/2514848620943889.

40 Annemarie Mol and Stacey Langwick offer exceptions to this, taking an ontological approach to understanding health and healing. Langwick, *Bodies, Politics, and African Healing*; Mol, *The Body Multiple*.

41 Alex Nading is another thinker whose work on entanglements and health has been particularly valuable for me. Alex's work focuses on the relationships between human health and the landscape, noting that changes to one reverberate through the other. This, he reveals, is the value of the concept of entanglement for understanding health. Alex M. Nading, *Mosquito Trails: Ecology, Health, and the Politics of Entanglement* (Berkeley: University of California Press, 2014).

42 Robert M. Jasmer, Payam Nahid, and Philip C. Hopewell, "Latent Tuberculosis Infection," *New England Journal of Medicine* 347, no. 23 (2002): 1860–66; Vinay Kumar and Stanley L. Robbins, *Robbins Basic Pathology*, 8th ed. (Philadelphia: Saunders/Elsevier, 2007); World Health Organization, "Tuberculosis," http://www.who.int/mediacentre/factsheets/fs104/en/index.html.

43 One study revealed that people who are repeatedly exposed to TB have a 22 percent higher infection rate than those who are less frequently exposed. N. Ahmed and S. E. Hasnain, "Molecular Epidemiology of Tuberculosis in India: Moving Forward with a Systems Biology Approach," *Tuberculosis* 91, no. 5 (2011): 407–13.

44 Cecil Slome and other medical directors had long understood TB to be rooted

in South Africa's political economy, which is key for understanding TB through a political-ecology framework. He explained, "The constant return of sick men from the towns is perpetuating the problem of tuberculosis . . . for they are reluctant to disclose their disease in the fear that they would be forced to receive therapy and give up their jobs. Further, these men, not having the continuous educational relationship with a health service tend, in spite of urban living, to retain their traditional beliefs in witchcraft and their opposition to modern therapy, both for themselves and their families." Slome, "Community Health in Rural Pholela," 285. Also see Kark and Steuart, *A Practice of Social Medicine*, 283–85.

The theory that tuberculosis came to rural areas from cities was (and continues to be) the reigning theory of how TB spread to rural areas in South Africa. In his landmark book *White Plague, Black Labor*, Randall Packard writes about the history of tuberculosis in South Africa as well as the history of scientific knowledge and government policy concerning tuberculosis. He argues that the mining industry's seemingly insatiable need for labor, combined with what appeared to be an inexhaustible supply of labor in the late nineteenth and early twentieth centuries, meant that mining companies offset the costs of tuberculosis by sending ill workers back to the Reserves to be cared for by their families. Randall M. Packard, *White Plague, Black Labor: Tuberculosis and the Political Economy of Health and Disease in South Africa* (Berkeley: University of California Press, 1989).

45 As Karen Barad writes, "Causal relations cannot be thought of as specific relations between isolated objects; rather causal relations necessarily entail a specification of the material apparatus that enacts an agential cut between determinately bounded and propertied entities within a phenomenon." Barad, *Meeting the Universe Halfway*, 18.

46 As I note in the introduction, illnesses, like the bodies that Annemarie Mol writes about in her work on the multiple bodies enacted through the diagnosis and treatment of atherosclerosis in a hospital in the Netherlands, offer, in the words of Stacey Langwick, "moments of ontological coordination," where worlds of health and healing become visible. Here Langwick describes Mol's work on arteriosclerosis. Langwick, *Bodies, Politics, and African Healing*, 23.

47 Mol, "A Reader's Guide to the 'Ontological Turn'—Part 4."

48 Here Langwick describes Mol's work on arteriosclerosis. Langwick, *Bodies, Politics, and African Healing*, 23.

49 I write about this for a more contemporary case of idliso in Neely, "An Object-Centered Ethnography for Global Health."

Conclusion: Social Medicine in the Age of Global Health

1 For example, see Vincanne Adams, Thomas E. Novotny, and Hannah Leslie, "Global Health Diplomacy," *Medical Anthropology* 27, no. 4 (2008): 315–23; Vincanne Adams, "Against Global Health: Arbitrating Science, Non-Science, and Nonsense through Health," in *Against Health: How Health Became a New Morality*, ed. Jonathan Metzl and Anna Kirkland (New York: NYU Press, 2010); Vincanne Adams, Nancy J. Burke, and Ian Whitmarsh, "Slow Research: Thoughts for a

Movement in Global Health," *Medical Anthropology* 33, no. 3 (2013): 179–97; Crystal Biruk, "Seeing Like a Research Project: Producing 'High-Quality Data' in AIDS Research in Malawi," *Medical Anthropology* 31, no. 4 (2012): 347–66; Betsey Brada, "'Not Here': Making the Spaces and Subjects of 'Global Health' in Botswana," *Culture, Medicine, and Psychiatry* 35, no. 2 (2011): 285–312; Johanna Crane, "Unequal 'Partners': AIDS, Academia, and the Rise of Global Health," *Behemoth: A Journal on Civilisation* 3, no. 3 (2010): 78–97; Johanna Crane, "Scrambling for Africa? Universities and Global Health," *The Lancet* 377, no. 9775 (2011): 1388–90; Craig R. Janes and Kitty K. Corbett, "Anthropology and Global Health," *Annual Review of Anthropology* 38 (2009): 167–83; Vinh-Kim Nguyen, *The Republic of Therapy: Triage and Sovereignty in West Africa's Time of AIDS* (Durham, NC: Duke University Press, 2010); James Pfeiffer and Mark Nichter, "What Can Critical Medical Anthropology Contribute to Global Health?," *Medical Anthropology Quarterly* 22, no. 4 (2008): 410–15; Matthew Sparke, "Unpacking Economism and Remapping the Terrain of Global Health," in *Global Health Governance: Transformations, Challenges and Opportunities amidst Globalization*, ed. Adrian Kay and Owain Williams (New York: Palgrave Macmillan, 2009); Claire L. Wendland, "Moral Maps and Medical Imaginaries: Clinical Tourism at Malawi's College of Medicine," *American Anthropologist* 114, no. 1 (2012): 108–22.

2   A lot of people have written about the ways in which HIV/AIDS is articulated through phenomena like witchcraft. This book is an argument against translating witchcraft into biomedical diseases. Nevertheless, this work is still valuable because it shows that some of the illness that presents under the broad category of "these diseases" is beyond the purview of biomedicine. For example, see Matthew Schoffeleers, "The AIDS Pandemic, the Prophet Billy Chisupe, and the Democratization Process in Malawi," *Journal of Religion in Africa* 29, no. 4 (1999): 404–41; Jonny Steinberg, *Sizwe's Test: A Young Man's Journey through Africa's AIDS Epidemic* (New York: Simon and Schuster, 2008).

Archival Sources

Rockefeller Archived Center (RAC)
    RFC: Rockefeller Foundation Collection
South African National Archives (SAB)
    GES: Secretary of Health
    VWN: Department of National Welfare, 1903–1972
    NTS: Secretary of Native Affairs, 1880–1975
University of the Witwatersrand Historical Papers (WHP)
    SAIRR: South African Institute for Race Relations Papers

Published Sources

Adams, Vincanne. "Against Global Health: Arbitrating Science, Non-Science, and Nonsense through Health." In *Against Health: How Health Became a New Morality*, edited by Jonathan Metzl and Anna Kirkland. New York: NYU Press, 2010.

Adams, Vincanne, ed. *Metrics: What Counts in Global Health*. Durham, NC: Duke University Press, 2016.

Adams, Vincanne, Nancy J. Burke, and Ian Whitmarsh. "Slow Research: Thoughts for a Movement in Global Health." *Medical Anthropology* 33, no. 3 (2013): 179–97.

Adams, Vincanne, Thomas E. Novotny, and Hannah Leslie. "Global Health Diplomacy." *Medical Anthropology* 27, no. 4 (2008): 315–23.

Agrawal, Arun, and Clark C. Gibson. "Enchantment and Disenchantment: The Role of Community in Natural Resource Conservation." *World Development* 27, no. 4 (1999): 629–49.

Ahmed, N., and S. E. Hasnain. "Molecular Epidemiology of Tuberculosis in India: Moving Forward with a Systems Biology Approach." *Tuberculosis* 91, no. 5 (2011): 407–13.

Ahmed, Sara. "Orientations Matter." In *New Materialisms: Ontology, Agency, and Politics*, edited by Diana Coole, 234–57. Durham, NC: Duke University Press, 2010.

Anderson, Ben, Matthew Kearnes, Colin McFarlane, and Dan Swanton. "On Assemblages and Geography." *Dialogues in Human Geography* 2, no. 2 (2012): 171–89.

Applegate, Elizabeth. "Introduction: Nutritional and Functional Roles of Eggs in the Diet." *Journal of the American College of Nutrition* 19, supp. 5 (2000): 495S–98S.

Ashforth, Adam. *Madumo: A Man Bewitched*. Chicago: University of Chicago Press, 2000.

Ashforth, Adam. *Witchcraft, Violence, and Democracy in South Africa*. Chicago: University of Chicago Press, 2005.

Bailey, Martha J., and Andrew Goodman-Bacon. "The War on Poverty's Experiment in Public Medicine: Community Health Centers and the Mortality of Older Americans." *NBER Working Paper* no. 20653. Boston: National Bureau of Economic Research, 2014.

Barad, Karen. *Meeting the Universe Halfway: Quantum Physics and the Entanglement of Matter and Meaning.* Durham, NC: Duke University Press, 2007.

Barad, Karen. "Posthumanist Performativity: Toward an Understanding of How Matter Comes to Matter." *Signs* 28, no. 3 (2003): 801–31.

Bauchspies, Wenda K., and Maria Puig de la Bellacasa. "Feminist Science and Technology Studies: A Patchwork of Moving Subjectivities. An Interview with Geoffrey Bowker, Sandra Harding, Anne Marie Mol, Susan Leigh Star and Banu Subramaniam." *Subjectivity* 28, no. 1 (2009): 334–44.

Beinart, William. *Twentieth-Century South Africa.* New York: Oxford University Press, 2001.

Bennett, Jane. *Vibrant Matter: A Political Ecology of Things.* Durham, NC: Duke University Press, 2009.

Biehl, João, and Adriana Petryna. *When People Come First: Critical Studies in Global Health.* Princeton, NJ: Princeton University Press, 2013.

Biruk, Crystal. *Cooking Data: Culture and Politics in an African Research World.* Durham, NC: Duke University Press, 2018.

Biruk, Crystal. "Seeing Like a Research Project: Producing 'High-Quality Data' in AIDS Research in Malawi." *Medical Anthropology* 31, no. 4 (2012): 347–66.

Biruk, Crystal, and Dana Prince. "'Subjects, Participants, Collaborators': Reading Community in Public Health Literature." *International Feminist Journal of Politics* 10, no. 2 (2008): 236–46.

Blaikie, Piers M., Harold C. Brookfield, and Bryant James Allen. *Land Degradation and Society.* New York: Methuen, 1987.

Bloor, David. *Knowledge and Social Imagery.* Chicago: University of Chicago Press, 1991.

Bowker, Geoffrey C., and Susan Leigh Star. *Sorting Things Out: Classification and Its Consequences.* Cambridge, MA: MIT Press, 2000.

Brada, Betsey. "'Not Here': Making the Spaces and Subjects of 'Global Health' in Botswana." *Culture, Medicine, and Psychiatry* 35, no. 2 (2011): 285–312.

Braun, Bruce. "Editorial: Querying Posthumanisms." *Geoforum* 35 (2004): 269–73.

Braun, Bruce, and Noel Castree. *Remaking Reality: Nature at the Millenium.* London: Routledge, 2005.

Breckenridge, Keith. *Biometric State.* Cambridge: Cambridge University Press, 2014.

Brenner, Neil. "Urban Governance and the Production of New State Spaces in Western Europe, 1960–2000." *Review of International Political Economy* 11, no. 3 (2004): 447–88.

Brotherton, P. Sean, and Vinh-Kim Nguyen. "Revisiting Local Biology in the Era of Global Health." *Medical Anthropology* 32, no. 4 (2013): 287–90.

Brown, Theodore M., and Elizabeth Fee. "Rudolf Carl Virchow: Medical Scientist, Social Reformer, Role Model." *American Journal of Public Health* 96, no. 12 (2006): 2104–5.

Bryant, A. T. *A History of the Zulu and Neighbouring Tribes*. Cape Town: C. Struik, 1964.

Bryant, A. T. *Zulu Medicine and Medicine-Men*. Cape Town: C. Struik, 1966.

Bryant, Raymond L. *The International Handbook of Political Ecology*. Cheltenham, UK: Edward Elgar, 2015.

Cahill, Caitlin, Farhana Sultana, and Rachel Pain. "Participatory Ethics: Politics, Practices, Institutions." *ACME: An International E-Journal for Critical Geographies* 6, no. 3 (2007): 304–18.

Callon, Michel, and Bruno Latour. "Don't Throw the Baby Out with the Bath School! A Reply to Collins and Yearley." *Science as Practice and Culture* 343 (1992): 368.

Carpenter, Kenneth J. "A Short History of Nutritional Science: Part 3 (1912–1944)." *Journal of Nutrition* 133, no. 10 (2003): 3023–32.

Carpenter, Kenneth J. "A Short History of Nutritional Science: Part 4 (1945–1985)." *Journal of Nutrition* 133, no. 11 (2003): 3331–42.

Cassel, John. "A Comprehensive Health Program among South African Zulus." In *Health, Culture, and Community: Case Studies of Public Reactions to Health Programs*, edited by Benjamin D. Paul and Walter B. Miller, 15–41. New York: Russell Sage Foundation, 1955.

Cassel, John. "Cultural Factors in the Interpretation of Illness." In *A Practice of Social Medicine: A South African Team's Experiences in Different African Communities*, edited by Sidney L. Kark and Guy W. Steuart, 238–44. Edinburgh: E. & S. Livingstone, 1962.

Castro, Eduardo Viveiros de. "Cosmological Deixis and Amerindian Perspectivism." *Journal of the Royal Anthropological Institute* 4, no. 3 (1998): 469–88.

Castro, Eduardo Batalha Viveiros de. "Exchanging Perspectives: The Transformation of Objects into Subjects in Amerindian Ontologies." *Common Knowledge* 10, no. 3 (2004): 463–84.

Cluver, Eustace Henry. *Public Health in South Africa*, 5th ed. Johannesburg: Central News Agency, 1948.

Cluver, Eustace Henry. *Social Medicine*. Johannesburg: Central News Agency, 1951.

"Commencement 2016: Biographies—H. Jack Geiger." *TuftsNow*, 2016. https://now .tufts.edu/commencement2016/biographies/geiger.

Commission on Native Affairs. *Report of the Native Affairs Commission Appointed to Enquire into the Working of the Provisions of the Natives (Urban Areas) Act Relating to the Use and Supply of Kaffir Beer*. Pretoria: Government Printing Office, 1942.

"Community Oriented Primary Care." *American Journal of Public Health* 92, no. 11 (2002).

Cope, Meghan. "Feminist Epistemology in Geography." In *Feminist Geography in Practice: Research and Methods*, edited by Pamela Moss. Oxford: Blackwell, 2002.

Craddock, Susan. *Compound Solutions: Pharmaceutical Alternatives for Global Health*. Minneapolis: University of Minnesota Press, 2017.

Crane, Johanna. *Scrambling for Africa: AIDS, Expertise, and the Rise of American Global Health Science*. Ithaca, NY: Cornell University Press, 2013.

Crane, Johanna. "Scrambling for Africa? Universities and Global Health." *The Lancet* 377, no. 9775 (2011): 1388–90.

Crane, Johanna. "Unequal 'Partners': AIDS, Academia, and the Rise of Global Health." *Behemoth: A Journal on Civilisation* 3, no. 3 (2010): 78–97.

Crang, Mike. "Qualitative Methods: Touchy, Feely, Look-See?" *Progress in Human Geography* 27, no. 4 (2003): 494–504.

Cronon, William. *Uncommon Ground: Rethinking the Human Place in Nature*. New York: W. W. Norton, 1996.

Dawson, Bertram Lord. "Interim Report on the Future Provision of Medical and Allied Services." London: Ministry of Health, Consultative Council on Medical and Allied Services, 1920.

de la Cadena, Marisol. *Earth Beings: Ecologies of Practice across Andean Worlds*. Durham, NC: Duke University Press, 2015.

de la Cadena, Marisol. "Indigenous Cosmopolitics in the Andes: Conceptual Reflections beyond 'Politics.'" *Cultural Anthropology* 25, no. 2 (2010): 334–70.

de Laet, Marianne, and Annemarie Mol. "The Zimbabwe Bush Pump: Mechanics of a Fluid Technology." *Social Studies of Science* 30, no. 2 (2000).

Deleuze, Gilles, and Félix Guattari. *Anti-Oedipus*. London: A&C Black, 2004.

Deleuze, Gilles, and Félix Guattari. *A Thousand Plateaus: Capitalism and Schizophrenia*. Translated by B. Massumi. Minneapolis: University of Minnesota Press, [1980] 1987.

Du Bois, W. E. B. *Black Reconstruction in America: Toward a History of the Part Which Black Folk Played in the Attempt to Reconstruct Democracy in America, 1860–1880*. London: Routledge, 2017.

Dubow, Saul. *Racial Segregation and the Origins of Apartheid in South Africa, 1919–36*. Basingstoke, UK: Palgrave Macmillan, 1989.

Dubow, Saul, and Alan Jeeves. *South Africa's 1940s: Worlds of Possibilities*. Cape Town: Double Storey, 2005.

England, Kim V. L. "Getting Personal: Reflexivity, Positionality, and Feminist Research." *Professional Geographer* 46, no. 1 (1994): 80–89.

Farmer, Paul. *AIDS and Accusation: Haiti and the Geography of Blame*, rev. ed. Berkeley: University of California Press, 2006.

Farmer, Paul. *Infections and Inequalities: The Modern Plagues*. Berkeley: University of California Press, 1999.

Farmer, Paul. "On Suffering and Structural Violence: A View from Below." *Daedalus* 125, no. 1 (1996): 261–83.

Farmer, Paul. *Pathologies of Power: Health, Human Rights, and the New War on the Poor*. Berkeley: University of California Press, 2005.

Farmer, Paul, Philippe Bourgois, Nancy Scheper-Hughes, Didier Fassin, Linda Green, H. K. Heggenhougen, Laurence Kirmayer, and Loïc Wacquant. "An Anthropology of Structural Violence 1." *Current Anthropology* 45, no. 3 (2004): 305–25.

Feierman, Steven. "Explaining Uncertainty in the Medical World of Ghaambo." *Bulletin of the History of Medicine* 74 (2000): 317–44.

Feierman, Steven. "Struggles for Control: The Social Roots of Health and Healing in Modern Africa." *African Studies Review* 28, nos. 2–3 (1985): 73–147.

Feierman, Steven, and John M. Janzen, eds. *The Social Basis of Health and Healing in Africa*. Berkeley: University of California Press, 1992.

Forsyth, Timothy. "Mountain Myths Revisited: Integrating Natural and Social Environmental Science." *Mountain Research and Development* 18, no. 2 (1998): 107–16.

Foster, Laura A. *Reinventing Hoodia: Peoples, Plants, and Patents in South Africa*. Seattle: University of Washington Press, 2017.

Foucault, Michel. *The Birth of the Clinic: An Archaeology of Medical Perception*. New York: Pantheon, 1973.

Foucault, Michel. *The History of Sexuality: An Introduction*. Translated by Robert Hurley. New York: Vintage, 1990.

Fox, F. William, and Douglas Back. "A Preliminary Survey of the Agricultural and Nutritional Problems of the Ciskei and Transkeian Territories with Special Reference to Their Bearing on the Recruiting of Labourers for the Gold Mining Industry." Johannesburg: Unpublished MS, 1943.

"Freedom Day Struggle Heroes: Steve Biko and Donald James Woods." *YouTube*, April 28, 2015. https://www.youtube.com/watch?v=cPHTxiDcW8o.

Fujimura, Joan H. "Crafting Science: Standardized Packages, Boundary Objects, and 'Translation.'" *Science as Practice and Culture* 168, no. 1992 (1992): 168–69.

Geiger, H. Jack. "Community-Oriented Primary Care: A Path to Community Development." *American Journal of Public Health* 92, no. 11 (2002): 1713–16.

Gibson-Graham, Julie-Kathy. "'Stuffed If I Know!': Reflections on Post-Modern Feminist Social Research." *Gender, Place and Culture* 1, no. 2 (1994): 205–24.

Gillman, Joseph, and Theodore Gillman. *Perspectives in Human Malnutrition: A Contribution to the Biology of Disease from a Clinical and Pathological Study of Chronic Malnutrition and Pellagra in the African*. New York: Grune and Stratton, 1951.

Gluckman, Henry. *Report of the National Health Services Commission on the Provision of an Organized National Health Service for All Sections of the People of the Union of South Africa, 1942–1944*. Pretoria: Government Printer, 1944.

Goldman, Mara J., Paul Nadasdy, and Matthew D. Turner. *Knowing Nature: Conversations at the Intersection of Political Ecology and Science Studies*. Chicago: University of Chicago Press, 2011.

Good, Byron J. *Medicine, Rationality and Experience: An Anthropological Perspective*. Cambridge: Cambridge University Press, 1993.

Greenhough, Beth. "Assembling an Island Laboratory." *Area* 43, no. 2 (2011): 134–38.

Gregory, Derek. *Geographical Imaginations*. Cambridge, MA: Blackwell, 1994.

Guthman, Julie. "Introducing Critical Nutrition: A Special Issue on Dietary Advice and Its Discontents." *Gastronomica* 14, no. 3 (2014): 1–4.

Guthman, Julie. "Opening Up the Black Box of the Body in Geographical Obesity Research: Toward a Critical Political Ecology of Fat." *Annals of the Association of American Geographers* 102, no. 5 (2012): 951–57.

Guthman, Julie. *Weighing In: Obesity, Food Justice, and the Limits of Capitalism*. Berkeley: University of California Press, 2011.

Guthman, Julie, and Becky Mansfield. "The Implications of Environmental Epigenetics: A New Direction for Geographic Inquiry on Health, Space, and Nature-Society Relations." *Progress in Human Geography* 37, no. 4 (2013): 486–504.

Guthman, Julie, and Becky Mansfield. "Nature, Difference, and the Body." In *The Routledge Handbook of Political Ecology*, edited by Tom Perreault, Gavin Bridge, and James McCarthy, 558–70. New York: Routledge, 2015.

Guyer, Jane I. "Household and Community in African Studies." *African Studies Review* 24, nos. 2–3 (1981): 87–138.

Guyer, Jane I., Naveeda Khan, Juan Obarrio, Caroline Bledsoe, Julie Chu, Souleymane Bachir Diagne, Keith Hart, Paul Kockelman, Jean Lave, and Caroline McLoughlin. "Introduction: Number as Inventive Frontier." *Anthropological Theory* 10, nos. 1–2 (2010): 36–61.

"H. Jack Geiger, MD, M Sci Hyg." Physicians for Human Rights, n.d. http://physicians forhumanrights.org/about/people/board-emeriti/h-jack-geiger.html.

Hammond-Tooke, W. D. *Rituals and Medicines: Indigenous Healing in South Africa.* Johannesburg: Ad. Donker, 1989.

Hammond-Tooke, W. D., and Isaac Schapera. *The Bantu-Speaking Peoples of Southern Africa*, 2nd ed. London: Routledge and Kegan Paul, 1974.

Haraway, Donna J. *The Companion Species Manifesto: Dogs, People, and Significant Otherness*, vol. 1. Chicago: Prickly Paradigm, 2003.

Haraway, Donna J. *Modest_Witness@Second_Millennium.Femaleman©_Meets_Oncomouse™: Feminism and Technoscience.* New York: Routledge, 1997.

Haraway, Donna J. *Primate Visions: Gender, Race, and Nature in the World of Modern Science.* New York: Psychology Press, 1989.

Haraway, Donna J. *Simians, Cyborgs, and Women: The Reinvention of Nature.* New York: Routledge, 1991.

Haraway, Donna J. "Situated Knowledges: The Science Question in Feminism and the Privilege of Partial Perspective." *Feminist Studies* 14, no. 3 (1988): 575–99.

Haraway, Donna J. *When Species Meet.* Minneapolis: University of Minnesota Press, 2008.

Harding, Sandra, ed. *Feminism and Methodology: Social Science Issues.* Bloomington: Indiana University Press, 1987.

Harding, Sandra. "Postcolonial and Feminist Philosophies of Science and Technology: Convergences and Dissonances." *Postcolonial Studies* 12, no. 4 (2009): 401–21.

Harding, Sandra. *The Science Question in Feminism.* Ithaca, NY: Cornell University Press, 1986.

Harding, Sandra. *Whose Science? Whose Knowledge? Thinking from Women's Lives.* Ithaca, NY: Cornell University Press, 1991.

Harley, J. Brian. "Deconstructing the Map." *Cartographica: The International Journal for Geographic Information and Geovisualization* 26, no. 2 (1989): 1–20.

Harley, J. Brian. "Maps, Knowledge, and Power." In *Geographic Thought: A Praxis Perspective*, edited by George L. Henderson and Marvin Waterstone, 129–48. Abingdon, UK: Routledge, 2009.

Harley, J. Brian. *The New Nature of Maps: Essays in the History of Cartography.* Baltimore: Johns Hopkins University Press, 2002.

Harries, Patrick. *Work, Culture, and Identity: Migrant Laborers in Mozambique and South Africa, c. 1860–1910.* Portsmouth, NH: Heinemann, 1994.

Hart, Gillian Patricia. *Disabling Globalization: Places of Power in Post-Apartheid South Africa.* Berkeley: University of California Press, 2002.

Hausermann, Heidi Eileen. "'I Could Not Be Idle Any Longer': Buruli Ulcer Treatment Assemblages in Rural Ghana." *Environment and Planning A* 47, no. 10 (2015): 2204–20.

Hayes-Conroy, Allison, and Jessica Hayes-Conroy. "Taking Back Taste: Feminism, Food and Visceral Politics." *Gender, Place and Culture* 15, no. 5 (2008): 461–73.

Henderson, Patricia C. *AIDS, Intimacy and Care in Rural Kwazulu-Natal: A Kinship of Bones.* Amsterdam: Amsterdam University Press, 2011.

Henderson, Patricia C. "The Vertiginous Body and Social Metamorphosis in a Context of HIV/AIDS." *Anthropology Southern Africa* 27, nos. 1–2 (2004): 43–53.

Henson, Ted. "Jack Geiger, MD, M.Sc., Scd." *We Are Public Health*, March 10, 2014. http://wearepublichealthproject.org/interview/jack-geiger/.

Heynen, Nik. "Bending the Bars of Empire from Every Ghetto for Survival: The Black Panther Party's Radical Antihunger Politics of Social Reproduction and Scale." *Annals of the Association of American Geographers* 99, no. 2 (2009): 406–22.

Heynen, Nikolas C. "The Scalar Production of Injustice within the Urban Forest." *Antipode* 35, no. 5 (2003): 980–98.

Holifield, Ryan. "Defining Environmental Justice and Environmental Racism." *Urban Geography* 22, no. 1 (2001): 78–90.

Holmes, Seth. *Fresh Fruit, Broken Bodies: Migrant Farmworkers in the United States.* Berkeley: University of California Press, 2013.

Howitt, Richard. "Scale as Relation: Musical Metaphors of Geographical Scale." *Area* 30, no. 1 (1998): 49–58.

Hunt, Sarah. "Ontologies of Indigeneity: The Politics of Embodying a Concept." *cultural geographies* 21, no. 1 (2014): 27–32.

Hunter, Mark. *Love in the Time of AIDS: Inequality, Gender, and Rights in South Africa.* Bloomington: Indiana University Press, 2010.

Hunter, Mark. "The Materiality of Everyday Sex: Thinking beyond 'Prostitution.'" *African Studies* 61, no. 1 (2002): 99–120.

"Interview with Karen Barad." In *New Materialism: Interviews and Cartographies*, edited by Rick Dolphijn and Iris van der Tuin, 48–70. Ann Arbor, MI: Open Humanities Press.

Isaacman, Allen. "Peasants and Rural Social Protest in Africa." *African Studies Review* 33, no. 2 (1990): 1–120.

Jackson, Paul, and Abigail H. Neely. "Triangulating Health toward a Practice of a Political Ecology of Health." *Progress in Human Geography* 39, no. 1 (2015): 47–64.

Jackson, Peter. *Maps of Meaning.* London: Routledge, 2012.

Janes, Craig R., and Kitty K. Corbett. "Anthropology and Global Health." *Annual Review of Anthropology* 38 (2009): 167–83.

Janzen, John M. *Ngoma: Discourses of Healing in Central and Southern Africa.* Berkeley: University of California Press, 1992.

Janzen, John M. "Therapy Management: Concept, Reality, Process." *Medical Anthropology Quarterly* 1, no. 1 (1987): 68–84.

Janzen, John M., and William Arkinstall. *The Quest for Therapy in Lower Zaire.* Berkeley: University of California Press, 1978.

Jasmer, Robert M., Payam Nahid, and Philip C. Hopewell. "Latent Tuberculosis Infection." *New England Journal of Medicine* 347, no. 23 (2002): 1860–66.

Jeeves, Alan, and J. S. Crush. *White Farms, Black Labor: The State and Agrarian Change in Southern Africa, 1910–50*. Portsmouth, NH: James Currey, 1997.

Jones, J. D. Rheinallt, Clement Martyn Doke, and D. F. Bleek. *Bushmen of the Southern Kalahari*. Johannesburg: University of the Witwatersrand Press, 1937.

Jones, J. D. Rheinallt, and Reinhold Friedrich Alfred Hoernlé. *The Union's Burden of Poverty*. Johannesburg: South African Institute of Race Relations, 1942.

Jones, J. D. Rheinallt, and Winifred Hoernlé. *At the Crossroads*. Johannesburg: South African Institute of Race Relations, 1953.

Jones, J. D. Rheinallt, and Ambrose Lynn Saffery. *Social and Economic Conditions of Native Life in the Union of South Africa. Findings of the Native Economic Commission, 1930–1932*. Johannesburg: University of the Witwatersrand Press, 1935.

Kagonyera, George Mondo. "Research and Innovations in Makerere University and Prospects for Strategic Partnerships between Makerere/Uganda and Unisa/South Africa." Kampala, Uganda: Makerere University, 2013.

Kanis, H. W. "Experiments in Social Medicine among Rural African Populations." In *Perspectives on the Health System: Economics of Health in South Africa*, edited by Gill Westcott and Francis Wilson. Johannesburg: Ravan, 1979.

Kark, J. D., and J. H. Abramson. "Sidney Kark's Contributions to Epidemiology and Community Medicine." *International Journal of Epidemiology* 32, no. 5 (2003): 882–84.

Kark, Sidney L. *Epidemiology and Community Medicine*. New York: Appleton-Century-Crofts, 1974.

Kark, Sidney L. "Health Centre Service." In *Social Medicine*, edited by E. H. Cluver, 661–700. Johannesburg: Central News Agency, 1951.

Kark, Sidney L. "Migrant Labour and Family Health." In *A Practice of Social Medicine: A South African Team's Experiences in Different African Communities*, edited by Sidney L. Kark and Guy W. Steuart, 194–209. Edinburgh: E. & S. Livingstone, 1962.

Kark, Sidney L. *The Practice of Community-Oriented Primary Health Care*. New York: Appleton-Century-Crofts, 1981.

Kark, Sidney L., and John Cassel. "The Pholela Health Centre: A Progress Report." *South African Medical Journal* 26, no. 6 (1952): 101–4.

Kark, Sidney L., and Emily Kark. "Epidemiological Considerations of Malnutrition in Rural African School Children." In *A Practice of Social Medicine: A South African Team's Experiences in Different African Communities*, edited by Sidney L. Kark and Guy W. Steuart, 220–32. Edinburgh: E. & S. Livingstone, 1962.

Kark, Sidney L., and Emily Kark. *Promoting Community Health: From Pholela to Jerusalem*. Johannesburg: University of the Witwatersrand Press, 1999.

Kark, Sidney L., and Guy W. Steuart. *A Practice of Social Medicine: A South African Team's Experiences in Different African Communities*. Edinburgh: E. & S. Livingstone, 1962.

Kelley, Robin D. G. "What Did Cedric Robinson Mean by Racial Capitalism?" *Boston Review*, January 12, 2017. http://bostonreview.net/race/robin-d-g-kelley-what-did-cedric-robinson-mean-racial-capitalism.

Kimura, Aya H., Charlotte Biltekoff, Jessica Mudry, and Jessica Hayes-Conroy. "Nutrition as a Project." *Gastronomica: The Journal of Critical Food Studies* 14, no. 3 (2014): 34–45.

King, Brian. "Political Ecologies of Disease and Health." In *The Routledge Handbook of Political Ecology*, edited by Tom Perreault, Gavin Bridge, and James McCarthy, 297–313. New York: Routledge, 2015.

King, Brian. "Political Ecologies of Health." *Progress in Human Geography* 34, no. 1 (2010): 38–55.

King, Brian. "Spatialising Livelihoods: Resource Access and Livelihood Spaces in South Africa." *Transactions of the Institute of British Geographers* 36, no. 2 (2011): 297–313.

Kobayashi, Audrey. "Coloring the Field: Gender, 'Race,' and the Politics of Fieldwork." *Professional Geographer* 46, no. 1 (1994): 73–80.

Krige, Eileen Jensen. *The Social System of the Zulus*, 3rd ed. Pietermaritzburg: Shuter and Shooter, 1957.

Kumar, Vinay, and Stanley L. Robbins. *Robbins Basic Pathology*, 8th ed. Philadelphia: Saunders/Elsevier, 2007.

Lambert, John. *Betrayed Trust: Africans and the State in Colonial Natal*. Scottsville: University of Kwazulu Natal Press, 1995.

Lampland, Martha. "False Numbers as Formalizing Practices." *Social Studies of Science* 40, no. 3 (2010): 377–404.

Lampland, Martha, and Susan Leigh Star. *Standards and Their Stories: How Quantifying, Classifying, and Formalizing Practices Shape Everyday Life*. Ithaca, NY: Cornell University Press, 2009.

Langwick, Stacey A. "Articulate(d) Bodies: Traditional Medicine in a Tanzanian Hospital." *American Ethnologist* 35, no. 3 (2008): 428–39.

Langwick, Stacey A. *Bodies, Politics, and African Healing: The Matter of Maladies in Tanzania*. Bloomington: Indiana University Press, 2011.

Latour, Bruno. *Reassembling the Social: An Introduction to Actor-Network-Theory*. Oxford: Oxford University Press, 2005.

Latour, Bruno. *We Have Never Been Modern*. Cambridge, MA: Harvard University Press, 2012.

Lefebvre, Henri. *The Production of Space*. Translated by Donald Nicholson-Smith. Oxford: Blackwell, 1991.

Lock, Margaret. *Encounters with Aging: Mythologies of Menopause in Japan and North America*. Berkeley: University of California Press, 1993.

Lock, Margaret. "The Tempering of Medical Anthropology: Troubling Natural Categories." *Medical Anthropology Quarterly* 15, no. 4 (2001): 487–92.

Lock, Margaret, and Patricia Kaufert. "Menopause, Local Biologies, and Cultures of Aging." *American Journal of Human Biology* 13, no. 4 (2001): 494–504.

Macmillan, William M. *Africa Beyond the Union*. Johannesburg: South African Institute of Race Relations, 1949.

Macmillan, William M. *Africa Emergent: A Survey of Social, Political, and Economic Trends in British Africa*. Harmondsworth, UK: Penguin, 1949.

Macmillan, William M. *The Road to Self-Rule: A Study in Colonial Evolution*. London: Faber and Faber, 1959.

Macmillan, William M. *The South African Agrarian Problem and Its Historical Development*. Witwatersrand: Central News Agency, 1919.

Macmillan, William M., and John Philip. *Bantu, Boer, and Briton: The Making of the South African Native Problem*, rev. ed. Oxford: Clarendon, 1963.

Mandala, Elias. "Feeding and Fleecing the Native: How the Nyasaland Transport System Distorted a New Food Market, 1890s–1920s." *Journal of Southern African Studies* 32, no. 3 (2006): 503–24.

Mansfield, Becky. "Environmental Health as Biosecurity: 'Seafood Choices,' Risk, and the Pregnant Woman as Threshold." *Annals of the Association of American Geographers* 102, no. 5 (2012): 969–76.

Mansfield, Becky. "Health as a Nature-Society Question." *Environment and Planning A* 40 (2008): 1015–19.

Mansfield, Becky. "Race and the New Epigenetic Biopolitics of Environmental Health." *BioSocieties* 7, no. 4 (2012): 352–72.

Mansfield, Becky. "The Social Nature of Natural Childbirth." *Social Science and Medicine* 66, no. 5 (2008): 1084–94.

Mansfield, Becky, and Julie Guthman. "Epigenetic Life: Biological Plasticity, Abnormality, and New Configurations of Race and Reproduction." *cultural geographies* 22, no. 1 (2015): 3–20. doi:10.1177/1474474014555659

Marston, Sallie A. "The Social Construction of Scale." *Progress in Human Geography* 24, no. 2 (2000): 219–42.

Marston, Sallie A., John Paul Jones III, and Keith Woodward. "Human Geography without Scale." *Transactions of the Institute of British Geographers* 30, no. 4 (2005): 416–32.

Marx, Anthony W. *Making Race and Nation: A Comparison of South Africa, the United States, and Brazil.* Cambridge: Cambridge University Press, 1998.

McDowell, Linda. "Doing Gender: Feminism, Feminists and Research Methods in Human Geography." *Transactions of the Institute of British Geographers* 17, no. 4 (1992): 399–416.

McFarlane, Colin, and Ben Anderson. "Thinking with Assemblage." *Area* 43, no. 2 (2011): 162–64.

McKay, Deirdre. "Negotiating Positionings: Exchanging Life Stories in Research Interviews." In *Feminist Geography in Practice: Research and Methods*, edited by Pamela Moss. Oxford: Blackwell, 2002.

McKeown, Thomas. "Determinants of Health." *Life* 60, no. 40 (1978): 3.

McMaster, Robert B., and Eric Sheppard. "Introduction: Scale and Geographic Inquiry." In *Scale and Geographic Inquiry: Nature, Society, and Method*, edited by Robert B. McMaster and Eric Sheppard, 1–22. Malden, MA: Blackwell, 2004.

Merchant, Carolyn. *The Death of Nature: Women, Ecology, and Scientific Revolution.* San Francisco: HarperSanFrancisco, 1981.

Mkhwanazi, Nolwazi. "Medical Anthropology in Africa: The Trouble with a Single Story." *Medical Anthropology* 35, no. 2 (2016): 193–202.

Mol, Annemarie. *The Body Multiple: Ontology in Medical Practice.* Durham, NC: Duke University Press, 2002.

Mol, Annemarie. "A Reader's Guide to the 'Ontological Turn'—Part 4." *Somatosphere: Science, Medicine, and Anthropology,* March 19, 2014. http://somatosphere.net/2014/a-readers-guide-to-the-ontological-turn-part-4.html/.

Mollett, Sharlene. "Mapping Deception: The Politics of Mapping Miskito and Gari-
    funa Space in Honduras." *Annals of the Association of American Geographers* 103, no. 5
    (2013): 1227–41.
Moore, Donald S. "Subaltern Struggles and the Politics of Place: Remapping Resis-
    tance in Zimbabwe's Eastern Highlands." *Cultural Anthropology* 13, no. 3 (1998):
    344–81.
Müller, Martin. "Assemblages and Actor-Networks: Rethinking Socio-Material Power,
    Politics and Space." *Geography Compass* 9, no. 1 (2015): 27–41.
Nading, Alex M. *Mosquito Trails: Ecology, Health, and the Politics of Entanglement.* Berke-
    ley: University of California Press, 2014.
Nast, Heidi J. "Women in the Field: Critical Feminist Methodologies and Theoretical
    Perspectives." *Professional Geographer* 46, no. 1 (1994): 54–66.
National Library of Medicine. "Community Health: A Model for the World." *Against
    the Odds,* n.d. https://apps.nlm.nih.gov/againsttheodds/exhibit/community_health
    /model_world.cfm.
Native Economic Commission. *Report of the Native Economic Commission 1930–1932.* Pre-
    toria: Government Printer, 1932.
Neely, Abigail H. "Entangled Agencies: Rethinking Causality and Health in Political-
    Ecology." *Environment and Planning E: Nature and Space* (2020). https://doi.org/10
    .1177251484862094389.
Neely, Abigail H. "*Hlonipha* and Health." *Africa.* 91, no. 3.
Neely, Abigail H. "Internal Ecologies and the Limits of Local Biologies: A Political
    Ecology of Tuberculosis in the Time of AIDS." *Annals of the Association of American
    Geographers* 105, no. 4 (2015): 791–805.
Neely, Abigail H. "Worlds in a Bottle: An Object-Centered Ethnography for Global
    Health." *Medicine Anthropology Theory* 6, no. 4 (2019): 127–41. doi.org/10.17157/mat6
    .4.642.
Neely, Abigail H., and Alex M. Nading. "Global Health from the Outside: The Promise
    of Place-Based Research." *Health and Place* 45 (2017): 55–63.
Neely, Abigail H., and Thokozile Nguse. "Relationships and Research Methods: En-
    tanglements, Intra-Actions, and Diffraction." In *The Routledge Handbook of Political
    Ecology,* edited by Tom Perrault, Gavin Bridge, and James McCarthy, 140–49. Lon-
    don: Routledge, 2015.
Ngubane, Harriet. *Body and Mind in Zulu Medicine: An Ethnography of Health and Disease in
    Nyuswa-Zulu Thought and Practice.* London: Academic Press, 1977.
Nguyen, Vinh-Kim. *The Republic of Therapy: Triage and Sovereignty in West Africa's Time of
    AIDS.* Durham, NC: Duke University Press, 2010.
Niehaus, Isak A., Eliazaar Mohlala, and Kally Shokane. *Witchcraft, Power, and Politics: Ex-
    ploring the Occult in the South African Lowveld.* London: Pluto, 2001.
Oswald, N. T. A. "A Social Health Service without Social Doctors." *Social History of
    Medicine* 4, no. 2 (1991): 295–315.
Packard, Randall M. "The 'Healthy Reserve' and the 'Dressed Native': Discourses on
    Black Health and the Language of Legitimation in South Africa." *American Ethnolo-
    gist* 16, no. 4 (1989): 686–703.

Packard, Randall M. "The Invention of the 'Tropical Worker': Medical Research and the Quest for Central African Labor on the South African Gold Mines, 1903–36." *Journal of Southern African Studies* 34, no. 2 (1993): 271–92.

Packard, Randall M. *White Plague, Black Labor: Tuberculosis and the Political Economy of Health and Disease in South Africa*. Berkeley: University of California Press, 1989.

Perreault, Tom, Gavin Bridge, and James McCarthy. *The Routledge Handbook of Political Ecology*. London: Routledge, 2015.

Pfeiffer, James, and Mark Nichter. "What Can Critical Medical Anthropology Contribute to Global Health?" *Medical Anthropology Quarterly* 22, no. 4 (2008): 410–15.

Pigg, Stacy Leigh. "The Credible and the Credulous: The Question of 'Villagers' Beliefs' in Nepal." *Cultural Anthropology* 11, no. 2 (1996): 160–201.

Pollock, Anne, and Banu Subramaniam. "Resisting Power, Retooling Justice: Promises of Feminist Postcolonial Technosciences." *Science, Technology, and Human Values* 41, no. 6 (2016): 951–66.

Posel, Dorrit. "How Do Households Work? Migration, the Household and Remittance Behaviour in South Africa." *Social Dynamics* 27, no. 1 (2001): 165–89.

Pulido, Laura. *Black, Brown, Yellow, and Left: Radical Activism in Los Angeles*. Berkeley: University of California Press, 2006.

Pulido, Laura. "Rethinking Environmental Racism: White Privilege and Urban Development in Southern California." *Annals of the Association of American Geographers* 90, no. 1 (2000): 12–40.

Robbins, Paul. *Political Ecology: A Critical Introduction*, 2nd ed. Malden, MA: Wiley-Blackwell, 2012.

Robinson, Cedric J. *Black Marxism: The Making of the Black Radical Tradition*. Chapel Hill: University of North Carolina Press, 2000.

Rocheleau, Dianne, Barbara Thomas-Slayter, and Esther Wangari. *Feminist Political Ecology: Global Issues and Local Experience*. New York: Routledge, 2013.

Rodney, Walter. *How Europe Underdeveloped Africa*. Washington, DC: Howard University Press, 1972.

Rose, Gillian. "Situating Knowledges: Positionality, Reflexivities and Other Tactics." *Progress in Human Geography* 21, no. 3 (1997): 305–20.

Scheper-Hughes, Nancy. *Death without Weeping: The Violence of Everyday Life in Brazil*. Berkeley: University of California Press, 1993.

Scheper-Hughes, Nancy. "Ire in Ireland." *Ethnography* 1, no. 1 (2000): 117–40.

Scherz, China. "Stuck in the Clinic: Vernacular Healing and Medical Anthropology in Contemporary Sub-Saharan Africa." *Medical Anthropology Quarterly* 32, no. 4 (2018): 539–55.

Schoffeleers, Matthew. "The AIDS Pandemic, the Prophet Billy Chisupe, and the Democratization Process in Malawi." *Journal of Religion in Africa* 29, no. 4 (1999): 404–41.

Schroeder, Richard A. *Shady Practices: Agroforestry and Gender Politics in the Gambia*. Berkeley: University of California Press, 1999.

Schumaker, Lyn. *Africanizing Anthropology: Fieldwork, Networks, and the Making of Cultural Knowledge in Central Africa*. Durham, NC: Duke University Press, 2001.

Scott, James C. *Seeing Like a State: How Certain Schemes to Improve the Human Condition Have Failed*. New Haven, CT: Yale University Press, 1998.

Scott, James C. *Weapons of the Weak: Everyday Forms of Peasant Resistance*. New Haven, CT: Yale University Press, 1985.

Shani, Michal, Harry H. X. Wang, Samuel Y. S. Wong, and Sian M. Griffiths. "International Primary Care Snapshots: Israel and China." *British Journal of General Practice* 65, no. 634 (2015): 250–51.

Shiva, Vandana. *Biopiracy: The Plunder of Nature and Knowledge*. Berkeley, CA: North Atlantic, 2016.

Showers, Kate. *Imperial Gullies: Soil Erosion and Conservation in Lesotho*. Athens: Ohio University Press, 2005.

Sidel, Victor W. "The Barefoot Doctors of the People's Republic of China." *New England Journal of Medicine* 286, no. 24 (1972): 1292–300.

Sigerist, Henry E. *Socialized Medicine in the Soviet Union*. New York: W. W. Norton, 1937.

Slome, Cecil. "Community Health in Rural Pholela." In *A Practice of Social Medicine: A South African Team's Experiences in Different African Communities*, edited by Sidney L. Kark and Guy W. Steuart, 269–91. Edinburgh: E. & S. Livingstone, 1962.

Soss, Joe. "Talking Our Way to Meaningful Explanations: A Practice-Centered View of Interviewing for Interpretive Research." In *Interpretation and Method: Empirical Methods and the Interpretive Trend*, edited by Dvorra Yarrow and Peregrine Schwartz-Shea, 193–214. New York: Routledge, 2015.

Sparke, Matthew. "Unpacking Economism and Remapping the Terrain of Global Health." In *Global Health Governance: Transformations, Challenges and Opportunities amidst Globalization*, edited by Adrian Kay and Owain Williams, 131–59. New York: Palgrave Macmillan, 2009.

Staeheli, Lynn A., and Victoria A Lawson. "Feminism, Praxis, and Human Geography." *Geographical Analysis* 27, no. 4 (1995): 321–38.

Star, Susan Leigh, and James R. Griesemer. "Institutional Ecology, 'Translations' and Boundary Objects: Amateurs and Professionals in Berkeley's Museum of Vertebrate Zoology, 1907–39." *Social Studies of Science* 19, no. 3 (1989): 387–420.

Steinberg, Jonny. *Sizwe's Test: A Young Man's Journey through Africa's AIDS Epidemic*. New York: Simon and Schuster, 2008.

Strathern, Marilyn. "Don't Eat Unwashed Lettuce." *American Ethnologist* 33, no. 4 (2006): 532–34.

Sultana, Farhana. "Reflexivity, Positionality and Participatory Ethics: Negotiating Fieldwork Dilemmas in International Research." *ACME: An International E-Journal for Critical Geographies* 6, no. 3 (2007): 374–85.

Sundberg, Juanita. "Masculinist Epistemologies and the Politics of Fieldwork in Latin Americanist Geography." *Professional Geographer* 55, no. 2 (2003): 180–90.

Susser, Mervyn. "Pioneering Community-Oriented Primary Care." *Bulletin of the World Health Organization* 77, no. 5 (1999): 436–38.

Swyngedouw, Erik. "Neither Global nor Local: 'Glocalization' and the Politics of

Scale." In *Space of Globalization: Reasserting the Power of the Local*, edited by Erik Swyngedouw, 115–36. New York: Guilford/Longman, 1997.

Swyngedouw, Erik, and Nikolas C. Heynen. "Urban Political Ecology, Justice and the Politics of Scale." *Antipode* 35, no. 5 (2003): 898–918.

Taylor, Peter J. *Unruly Complexity: Ecology, Interpretation, Engagement.* Chicago: University of Chicago Press, 2010.

Thompson, Leonard Monteath. *A History of South Africa*, 3rd ed. New Haven, CT: Yale University Press, 2001.

Tilley, Helen. *Africa as a Living Laboratory: Empire, Development, and the Problem of Scientific Knowledge, 1870–1950.* Chicago: University of Chicago Press, 2011.

Todd, Zoe. "An Indigenous Feminist's Take on the Ontological Turn: 'Ontology' Is Just Another Word for Colonialism." *Journal of Historical Sociology* 29, no. 1 (2016): 4–22.

Tollman, S. M., and W. M. Pick. "Roots, Shoots, but Too Little Fruit: Assessing the Contribution of COPC in South Africa." *American Journal of Public Health* 92, no. 11 (2002): 1725–28.

Trostle, James A. *Epidemiology and Culture.* New York: Cambridge University Press, 2005.

Turner, Matthew. "Drought, Domestic Budgeting and Wealth Distribution in Sahelian Households." *Development and Change* 31, no. 5 (2000): 1009–35.

Vaughan, Megan. *The Story of an African Famine: Gender and Famine in Twentieth-Century Malawi.* New York: Cambridge University Press, 1987.

Walker, Cherryl, ed. *Women and Gender in Southern Africa to 1945.* Cape Town: David Philip, 1990.

Wendland, Claire L. *A Heart for the Work: Journeys through an African Medical School.* Chicago: University of Chicago Press, 2010.

Wendland, Claire L. "Moral Maps and Medical Imaginaries: Clinical Tourism at Malawi's College of Medicine." *American Anthropologist* 114, no. 1 (2012): 108–22.

Whatmore, Sarah. *Hybrid Geographies: Natures, Cultures, Spaces.* London: SAGE, 2002.

Whatmore, Sarah. "Materialist Returns: Practising Cultural Geography in and for a More-Than-Human World." *cultural geographies* 13, no. 4 (2006): 600–609.

Willey, Angela. "A World of Materialisms: Postcolonial Feminist Science Studies and the New Natural." *Science, Technology, and Human Values* 41, no. 6 (2016): 991–1014.

Williams, Raymond. "Ideas of Nature." In *Nature: Critical Concepts in the Social Sciences*, vol. 1: *Thinking the Natural*, edited by David Inglis, John Bone, and Rhoda Wilkie, 47–62. London: Routledge, 2005.

Wilson, Monica. *Reaction to Conquest: Effects of Contact with Europeans on the Pondo of South Africa.* London: Oxford University Press, 1936.

Wolfe, Patrick. *Settler Colonialism and the Transformation of Anthropology.* London: Cassell, 1999.

Wolpe, Harold. "Capitalism and Cheap Labour-Power in South Africa: From Segregation to Apartheid." *Economy and Society* 1, no. 4 (1972): 425–56.

World Health Organization. "Tuberculosis." http://www.who.int/mediacentre /factsheets/fs104/en/index.html.

Wylie, Diana. *Starving on a Full Stomach: Hunger and the Triumph of Cultural Racism in Modern South Africa*. Charlottesville: University Press of Virginia, 2001.

Yach, D., and S. M. Tollman. "Public Health Initiatives in South Africa in the 1940s and 1950s: Lessons for a Post-Apartheid Era." *American Journal of Public Health* 83, no. 7 (1993): 1043–50.

INDEX

Page numbers followed by *f* indicate figures.

causality: Barad on phenomena and, 144n45; entangled, 102–4; ontological multiplicity and, 97–98; tuberculosis vs. *idliso* and, 86, 95–96
chicken coops, 69
China, 7
Cluver, Eustace, 20–21, 138n11
Columbia Point Community Health Center (now Geiger-Gibson Community Health Center), Boston, xiii
community, defining and mapping of, 22–23, 120n23
community-oriented primary care (COPC): about, ix, 3–4; community as organizing feature of, 22–23; cooperatives and, 54; health center model, 19; quantitative social science and, 29; seeing like a health center, 37–40; worldwide spread of, xiii–xv. *See also* Pholela Community Health Centre
conversion stories, 89–90
cooperatives, 53–54
Craddock, Susan, 142n35
Crenshaw, Kimberlee, 128n37
cultural determinism, 88

Dart, Raymond, 118n11
Dawson Report (UK), 6
de Laet, Marianne, 54
Deleuze, Gilles, 112n24, 127n22
Delta Community Health Center, Mound Bayou, MS, xiii, 54
demonstration gardens, 64–67
Designated Area: map, 24f; stepwise expansion of, 24–27, 121n29, 137n7
development schemes, South Africa, 18–20
diffraction, 15–16

employment by PCHC, 72–73
England, Kim, 50, 126n17
entanglements, more-than-human: Barad's "phenomena" and, 143n39;

global health and entangled causality, 102–4; health as, 93–95; ontological multiplicity, 97–98, 140n29; scientific logics and, 102; social life and, 5, 80, 82, 94, 96, 98, 101; tuberculosis, *idliso*, and, 80, 96; witchcraft illnesses and, 91–92. *See also* relationships and relationality

families: body linked to community and nation by, 31; Kark on, 123n47; political economy and, 32; preservation of, 31–32
family files, 29–33
Farmer, Paul, 74, 100, 123n49, 134n67
Feierman, Steven, 110n18, 137n6, 139n19
feminist research methods, 15–16, 45, 49–50
feminist science studies, 12–13, 15–16, 91, 114n30, 143n39
food: "bad," 1–2; eggs, 69–70; food-serving protocols, 134n63; milk and powdered milk, 70–73, 85; prescriptions of, 66, 71–72, 77, 83, 136n77. *See also* gardens; nutrition
Fox, F. William, 59–60, 129n9

Gale, George, xiii–xiv
gardens: crop diversity, 67; demonstration gardens, 64–67; *intelezi* in the garden, 2, 3f, 4; vegetable gardens, 52–53, 64–68
Geiger, Jack, ix–xv
Geiger-Gibson Community Health Center, Boston, xiii
Gibson, Clark, 22–23
Gibson-Graham, J.-K., 49
global health, xv, 8, 101–4
Gluckman, Harry, 19
Goldman, Mara, 132n31
Good, Byron, 31
"Grow and Eat More Vegetables" campaign (PCHC), 52–53, 64–68
Guattari, Félix, 112n24, 127n22

Guthman, Julie, 113n25
Guyer, Jane, 23–24, 29

Haraway, Donna, 15, 57, 128n37
Harding, Sandra, 57, 115n35, 128n37
health center model. *See* community-oriented primary care; Pholela Community Health Centre
health education: household survey and, 46; nutrition program and, 64, 78; PCHC and, 3, 5–6, 17, 100; tuberculosis, *idliso*, and, 87–88
"Health Policy in Relation to Nutrition Needs" report, 131n21
Hebrew University, Israel, xiv
Heynen, Nik, 132n34
HIV/AIDS, 100, 102–3
Hlabeni typhoid outbreak, 33–37, 35f, 38–39
hlonipha-related milk prohibitions, 70–71, 85
Hoernlé, Winifred, 20
homesteads: definition of, 23–24; mapping of, 22–23; program for remaking, 51–55; return to, 101–2. *See also* gardens
household surveys, PCHC: defining the household, 23–25, 121n24; quantitative social science and, 25–29, 26f
Hunt, Sarah, 14
Hunter, Mark, 12

idliso: about, 90–93; as entanglement, 93–94; Khanyisile case, cultural determinism, and, 85–88; ontological multiplicity, limits of health center practice, and, 97–98; PCHC rejection of, 88–90; Thembisa case, political ecology, and, 82–84; treatment, 86–87. *See also* tuberculosis
illnesses: categories of, 10; kwashiorkor, 15, 72; "psychosocial," 110n19; syphilis, 30–32; youth and "these diseases," 102–4. See also *idliso*; malnutrition; tuberculosis; witchcraft illnesses
imithi. See *umuthi/imithi*

Institute for Family and Community Health (IFCH), University of Natal Medical School, xii, 117n7, 118n11
intelezi, 2, 3f, 4, 13, 92
intersectionality, 128n37
intra-action, 15–16, 94
inyanga/izinyanga (herbalists): about, 126n9; *idliso* and, 83, 85–89, 93; questions about seeing, 46
isangoma/izangoma (diviners): about, 10, 126n9; annual protection ritual, 92; entanglement and, 94; *idliso* and, 86, 89, 94; *intelezi* and, 13
Israel, xiii, xiv, 107n4

Jali, Edward, 17, 21, 37, 59
Janzen, John, 137n6, 139n19

Kark, Emily: arrival in Pholela, 7, 17; family files and, 30–32; IFCH and, xii; in Israel, xiv; nutrition and, 58; racial capitalism and, 74; relationships and, 43, 49–50; training, 20–21
Kark, Sidney: arrival in Pholela, 7, 17; Bantu Nutrition Survey and, 21, 59, 117n17; family files and, 30–32; on family situation, 123n47; on household definition, 121n24; IFCH and, xii; investigated as communist, 136n77; in Israel, xiv; Ministry of Health and, 21, 118n11; NUSAS and, 119n15; nutrition and, 58; racial capitalism and, 74; relationships and, 43, 49–50; training, 20–21; on tuberculosis case, 83
Kelley, Robin D. G., 60
Kobayashi, Audrey, 50
Kupat Holim Health Insurance Institution, Israel, 107n4
kwashiorkor, 15, 72

labor: migrant, 10; nutrition and labor regimes, 59–64
Lampland, Martha, 47–48, 125n8
land inequities, 8–9, 133n61

Langwick, Stacey, 13, 80, 90, 98, 108n9, 114n29, 115n32, 139n19, 144n46
Latour, Bruno, 55, 112n24, 136n2
Law, John, 112n24
livelihoods: embodied, 77; employment by PCHC and, 73; gendered, 9–10, 32; household surveys and, 23–28; nutrition and, 58–64, 67–68; outbreak maps and, 36, 38; political ecology and, 11–12; political economy of, 74–77; racial capitalism and, 6, 98. *See also* social life
local biologies, 114n30

Makerere University Medical School, Uganda, xiv
malnutrition, 21, 27, 53, 58–60, 63–64. *See also* nutrition
Mandela, Nelson, xii
Mansfield, Becky, 113n25, 135n70
mapping: of community and homesteads, 22–23; of typhoid outbreak, 34–36, 35*f*
market dependencies, national and global, 76–77
markets, local, 67–68
Marston, Sallie, 31
maternal and child welfare program (PCHC), 46–47
McKeown, Thomas, 6–7
medical pluralism, 12, 94, 104, 114n29
medicine, scientific. *See* biomedicine
migrant laborers, 9–10
milk and powdered milk, 70–73, 85
Ministry of Health, South Africa, 21, 118n11
Mkhwanazi, Nolwazi, 28–29
Mol, Annemarie, 54, 93, 98, 115n32, 142n37, 143n40, 144n46
Moore, Donald, 43
Mound Bayou, MS, xiii, 54

Nadasdy, Paul, 132n31
Nading, Alex, 143n41
National Health Services Commission, 19, 117n17

National Nutrition Council, 129n7
National Union of South African Students (NUSAS), 119n15
Native Affairs Commission Reports, 117n17
Native Economic Commission Report, 117n17
Native Reserves, *xf*, 8, 60
Natives Land Act (1913), 8
Ngubane, Harriet, 110n18
Nguse, Thokozile, 2*f*, 14
nonhumans. *See* assemblages; entanglements, more-than-human; relationships and relationality
nutrition: Bantu Nutrition Survey, 21, 59, 61, 117n17; cooking instructions, 66; food prescriptions, 66, 71–72, 77, 83, 136n77; "Grow and Eat More Vegetables" campaign, 52–53, 64–68; "Health Policy in Relation to Nutrition Needs" report, 131n21; labor, racial capitalism, and nutrition science, 59–64; macronutrients, 64; malnutrition, 21, 27, 53, 58–60, 63–64; micronutrients, 53, 64; National Nutrition Council, 129n7; nutrients in nutrition science, 62; official nutritional guidelines, 62–63; political ecology of, 73–78; political economy and, 58–59, 76–77; protein consumption/milk program, 69–73

objectivity, 57
ontological coordination, 13, 98, 115n32, 144n46
ontological multiplicity, 97–98, 140n29

"perspectives" as ontological, 140n29
phenomena and entanglements, 143n39
Phillips, Harry, 108n8
Phola, South Africa, 9*f*; in 1930s, 8–10; maps, *xf*, *xif*. *See also specific topics, such as* Designated Area
Pholela Community Health Centre (PCHC): community mapping and de-

fining the household, 22–24; conventional story of, 7–8; conversion stories, 89–90; "correct" and misleading answers, 46–47; as employer, 72–73; family files and qualitative analysis, 29–33; "Grow and Eat More Vegetables" campaign, 52–53, 64–68; history of, 3; HIV/AIDS clinic, 100; household surveys and quantitative social science, 25–29; limits of health center practice, 97–98; map, xif; maternal and child welfare program, 46–47; as model, xiii–xv, 4; reputation of, ix; resident participation, importance of, 42; roots of, 18–21; seeing like a health center, 37–40; specialization vs. primary care and, 99–100; statistical measurement and scales of analysis, 17–18; success of, 3–4, 17–18, 28, 47; typhoid outbreak control efforts, 33–37, 35f, 38–39. *See also* community-oriented primary care; nutrition; relationships and relationality; tuberculosis

pit latrines, 51, 79

pluralism, medical, 12, 94, 104, 114n29

political ecology: as approach, 10–12; Blaikie and Brookfield's soil erosion study, 75; global health and, 104; of health, 75–76; nutrition and, 73–78; tuberculosis, *idliso*, and, 82–84, 87

political economy: family and, 32; of livelihoods, 76–77; nutrition and, 58–59; PCHC and, 32; political ecology and, 11; tuberculosis and, 95–96, 143n44. *See also* racial capitalism

positionality, 49–50

practices, as concept, 93, 142n37

precision vs. accuracy, 126n13

prescriptions of food, 66, 71–72, 77, 83, 136n77

primary care, 99–100. *See also* community-oriented primary care

Prince, Dana, 120n23

protein consumption, 69–73

"psychosocial" illnesses, 110n19

purchasing habits, 71

qualitative social science, 20, 29–33, 37

quantitative social science, 25–29, 26f, 48–49

racial capitalism: apartheid and, 11–12, 60–61, 130n17; concept of, 6, 60–61; intervention difficulty, 52; landscapes and, 74; mediated by the health center, 77; nutrition, labor and, 60–64; political ecology and, 11–12, 77; South Africa and, 61; women's agriculture and men's low-wage labor, 10

Radebe, Gcina, xiv

reflexivity, 49–50, 125n6

relational ontologies, 90–91

relationships and relationality: assemblages and, 51–56, 112n24; become a researcher and, 43–45; biomedicine and, 11; feminist science studies and, 13; homestead remaking program and, 51–55; *intelezi* and, 13; PCHC and influence of participants' answers, 45–48; replicability vs. complexity and richness and, 48–50; science and, 57; social medicine and, 4–5, 56–57; tuberculosis and, 96. *See also* entanglements, more-than-human

replicability, 48–49

Rhodes-Livingston Institute (RLI), 56–57

richness, 49

rights, human, 7

Robinson, Cedric, 11, 60–61

Rodney, Walter, 61

Rose, Gillian, 56

Salber, Eva, 108n8

scale: hierarchical framework, 31; political ecology of health and, 75–76; social construction of, 31; statistical measurement and multiscalar practice, 18; typhoid outbreak and, 38–39

Schumaker, Lyn, 56–57
science: entanglements vs. scientific log-
    ics, 102; intersectionality and, 128n37;
    relationships and, 57. *See also* biomedi-
    cine; quantitative social science
Scotch, Norm, xiv
Scott, James, 18, 27–28, 47–48, 125n8
seed cooperatives, 53–54
Shiva, Vandana, 13–14
Shriver, Sargent, xii–xiii
Sigerist, Henry, 6
Slome, Cecil, 68, 108n8, 143n44
social life: assemblages and, 56, 112n24;
    entangled more-than-human relation-
    ships and, 5, 80, 82, 94, 96, 98, 101; fam-
    ily files, qualitative social science, and,
    29–33; feminist science studies and,
    114n30; global health and, 29, 102, 104;
    the household and, 24; *idliso* and, 90;
    nutrition and, 58–59, 64, 76; outbreak
    maps and, 36; race and, 63, 74, 77, 98;
    seeing like a health center and, 37–39;
    social medicine and, 7, 11–14, 43, 46, 77,
    80, 98, 101; social-sciences understand-
    ing of, 6, 18; tuberculosis and, 95–98;
    who or what counts as social, 55; witch-
    craft and, 81–82, 94, 98. *See also* liveli-
    hoods; relationships and relationality
social medicine: conventional story of,
    6–8; defined, ix; primary care, impor-
    tance of, 99–100; relationality and,
    4–5; what counts as social, 55. *See
    also* community-oriented primary
    care; Pholela Community Health
    Centre
social science: biomedicine and, 31,
    37–38, 56, 114n30; qualitative, 20,
    29–33, 37; quantitative, 24–29, 26f
social welfare programs, South Africa,
    18–20
Society of Medical Conditions, 119n15
South Africa: Ministry of Health, 21,
    118n11; nutrition science and, 63; racial
    capitalism and the "worker problem,"

61; social welfare programs, 18–20. *See
    also* apartheid; racial capitalism
South African Institute for Race Rela-
    tions (SAIRR), 21, 119n14, 129n7
South African Student Organization
    (SASO), 119n15
specialization vs. primary care, 99–100
standardization, 46, 48–49, 57, 125n8
Star, Susan Leigh, 47–48, 125n8
Stein, Zina, 108n8
Steuart, Guy, 108n8
Strathern, Marilyn, 56
Student Medical Council, 119n15
Subramaniam, Banu, 128n37
Susser, Mervyn, xiv, 108n8
symmetrical analysis, 80
syphilis, 30–32

Todd, Zoe, 140–41n29
traditional healing: biomedicine combined
    with, 10, 12–13; as fraught term, 108n9
tuberculosis (TB): Cluver on social struc-
    ture and, 138n11; as entanglement, 96;
    having both *idliso* and, 139n17; Khany-
    isile case, cultural determinism, and,
    85–88; *Mycobacterium tuberculosis*, 87,
    95; ontological multiplicity, limits of
    health center practice, and, 97–98;
    PCHC rejection of *idliso* and, 79–80,
    88–90; PCHC's failures in, 79–80; po-
    litical economy, entanglement, and,
    95–96; rates of, 79, 82, 140n25; Them-
    bisa case, political ecology, and, 82–84;
    treatment, 86; vaccine search, 142n35.
    See also *idliso*
Turner, Matthew, 132n31
typhoid outbreak control efforts, 33–37,
    35f, 38–39

Uganda, xiv
umthakathi/abathakathi (witchcraft prac-
    titioners): about, 10, 79; *idliso* and, 79,
    85, 87–88, 91–94; power of, 81. *See also*
    witchcraft illnesses